Memoirs

of

Miracles

by

"Uncle Tim" Mondy

Memoirs of Miracles by Tim Mondy

ISBN-13: 978-0-6151-9877-4

Copyright © 2008 by Tim Mondy

Published by: Tim Mondy

Dedication

This book is dedicated to those who battle the dreaded diseases collectively known as cancer.

Table of Contents

Forward

I am unsure why God allowed me to chronicle the events, which have comprised Ryan's battle with brain cancer. I stand humbled in His presence as I share the account of a truly incredible little boy.

A very special thank you is due Mrs. Marsha Humphrey for her extraordinary ability to refine my untrained words into an intelligible story.

As I have spoken with my brother Chris over the many months detailed in this work, I have tried to formulate this forward. That has been no easy task as there are too many people to recognize publicly one at a time.

For brevity sake, I would like to thank all of the staff at Arkansas Children's Hospital who have helped care for Ryan. The knowledge of these people is surpassed only by their compassion for children. Their love of children shows in their determined struggle to defeat the illnesses which plague these little ones.

Chris and Andrea have spent a tremendous amount of time in Little Rock, Arkansas, with Ryan over a span of several months. Chris wanted to say a special thank you to our mother, Nonna, for her willingness to stay at the hospital and the Ronald McDonald House for weeks on end to help care for Ryan.

While Nonna sat at the hospital with Ryan, Andrea's mother, Carnell Beck, stayed with her granddaughter because Andrea's brother, Steve, was serving in our country's military. Much of the time documented herein, Steve was stationed in Iraq. They could not stay at the hospital, but they helped wage the battle for Ryan as they continually prayed and requested those around them to do the same.

The remainder of our family has all been instrumental in lending aid and support during an extremely trying time and for that I know Chris and Andrea have been very touched.

I would also like to acknowledge the staff at the Little Rock Ronald McDonald House. They have grown to love and admire Ryan on his many trips to the hospital. The time he spent residing at the house during his chemotherapy and radiation was such a blessing to Chris and Andrea.

A special thank you is due everyone who has helped share Ryan's story with others. Every entry in the CaringBridge guestbook has been read and every one of the entries has touched the hearts of our family. To realize there were people all around the world who were supporting our family in prayer has helped us survive even the most difficult times.

Much strength has been gained from the congregation I pastor, the First Church of the Nazarene in Centralia, Illinois. The members of the congregation have prayed for our entire family through this time. They have cared for my immediate family, providing transportation, meals, and financial support as needed. Their loving support has been crucial at many points along this journey. I am ever grateful for all of the care.

Lastly, I would like to thank my wife, Laura, for all of her support and assistance as this work became a reality. She has been extremely generous in taking on extra responsibilities around our home so I could be available when my brother and his family needed me. She has been my sounding board and my confidant. When I needed to talk about the information I should or should not include, Laura has always been willing to help. Without her encouragement, I might never have gotten these words on paper.

As I began to write this book, I had two goals in mind. First, I wanted to share the incredibly inspirational story of Ryan's battle with this dread disease. The second goal was much more important to me. I wanted give God all of the glory and honor for what He has done through this time. There have been many instances throughout the writing process when I became convinced the book was completed. God has continued to prolong the process until He said it was finished. I have done my best to be faithful to these two goals, even in the times that I did not wish to continue writing. To God be all of the glory and honor for the miracles He has wrought in our family.

Uncle Tim

The First 48 Hours

As the phone rang, I reached to answer it. Caller I.D. told me it was my mom on the line. "Hi, Mom, what's up?"

When she spoke, the hitch in her voice immediately let me know something was wrong. "They found a mass on Ryan's brain and they're flying him by helicopter to the Arkansas Children's Hospital in Little Rock."

I stammered for a few seconds not knowing what to say. Finally, after what seemed an eternity, "What did you say?" came out of my mouth.

"Chris called to talk to your dad a few minutes ago. I knew something was up when I answered the phone and he wouldn't talk to me. He asked for your dad. Your dad went pale while they talked and I knew something bad had happened. Ryan went to the doctor today and they did a CT scan. They found a large mass on his brain. He is on the way to Little Rock right now; they are airlifting him by helicopter. Your dad and I are going to the hospital as quick as we can get our things together."

Ryan was my six-year-old nephew, the son of my brother Chris. Mom told me that she did not know any more details. She cut the conversation short and said she had to go so they could finish packing. Before she hung up the phone, she promised to let me know if she heard anything else.

I looked at the clock and it was almost 4:00 p.m. My wife and I were supposed to go out that night, but she had gone to run a few errands before we went. I tried to call her cell phone, but she didn't answer. I was not sure what to do, so I called Ryan's mom, Andrea, to ask her what had happened.

Andrea answered her phone, "I can't talk right now. Chris will call you back," and she hung up on me.

"That was rude," I thought to myself. The abrupt disconnect really made me wonder what was happening in Arkansas. I would have hopped into the car and gone to the hospital to see what was going on, but I lived in Illinois, hours away from Chris and Andrea. They were sitting in a doctor's office somewhere in northwest Arkansas. As it was, I lived too far away from them to get to the hospital; so, I sat back in my chair and tried to read something to keep myself occupied while I waited for Chris to call.

About fifteen minutes later, Chris returned my call. His voice sounded strained and anxious. I could hear his nervousness. As I listened to him, I must have gone ghostly white. He jumped into an explanation, which painted a picture that I had never anticipated viewing.

"Ryan had a sinus infection last week and he took a round of antibiotics for it. He finished the medicine, but he still had a headache. Andrea called the doctor's office yesterday and they renewed the prescription for more antibiotics. I was supposed to pick the prescription up last night on the way home from work, but I forgot. When we got up this morning, Ryan had a bad headache, so Andrea decided to take him in to see the doctor. We thought it was just another sinus headache, so I went on to work while Andrea took Ryan to the doctor's office."

So far, I was not surprised. Ryan had suffered from sinus trouble his entire life. While their family had lived in Utah, Ryan continually suffered from nosebleeds due to the dry air. He had also suffered from recurrent sinus infections the entire time they lived there. I wondered how they had made the jump from sinus headache to a mass on his brain.

Chris continued, "The doctor checked inside Ryan's ears and looked up his nose and everything seemed okay, but when he checked Ryan's eyes he saw a bulging of the optical discs and became concerned. The doctor asked Andrea if glaucoma ran in the family and when she told him that it did not he told her that he would like to have a CT scan performed on Ryan's head. Andrea told him to go ahead, so he called the hospital to schedule the test. He got the test scheduled for about 2:30 this afternoon. Andrea called me and asked me to meet them at the hospital for the CT scan. That was about 11:30 this morning while I was at lunch, but I told her I would finish the important stuff and meet her there."

He had finally started getting to the crux of the matter. I interrupted him for a moment. "What are optical discs, and why were they bulging?"

Testily, he replied, "I am not sure what they are, it has something to do with the optic nerve and extra pressure inside the head. May I continue now?"

"I was just asking a simple question," I meekly retorted. I didn't want to press the issue, so I dropped the matter. I figured I could get more information later if I really needed to know more about optical discs.

"I left the office about 1:30 to get to the hospital in time for the test, but at about 1:45, Andrea called while I was on the way to the hospital and told me that the test was done."

He paused for a moment and I wondered to myself why they would have done the test so quickly. As a pastor, I had spent a fair amount of time around hospitals. I had sat with families for hours while they waited to have tests like this one run. I knew that if the doctor scheduled a test time for 2:30 p.m., a patient was usually fortunate if he or she was out of the test by 5:00 p.m. Apparently, Chris had the same question, because after he had paused for a few seconds he began to talk again. As he started to speak, I noticed more of a quaver in his voice.

"When she told me that Ryan had been worked in early for the test I got concerned. I haven't heard of many CT scans performed an hour early, unless there is something seriously in question. I told Andrea that I was on my way to the hospital and I would be there as quickly as I could."

"I guess one doesn't have to be a pastor to become concerned when medical tests are rushed," I thought to myself. Aloud, I gave a slight assent to his comment, "I understand why you became concerned. They don't usually rush tests."

After a long pause, Chris' words began to slowly flow, as he continued his tale. It was as if he were remembering the details of some macabre nightmare. He didn't wish to remember any more details, but it was essential. I raptly hung on every word he spoke. I wished I could drag the story out quicker, but I felt I needed to let him tell the story in his own way.

"After I got to the hospital, I found my way to the CT waiting room. When I walked into the room, Ryan was lying with his head on Andrea's lap, watching TV. I sat down and waited with them for about ten minutes before the doctor called the nurses' station and asked to speak to Andrea. The doctor was still at the clinic, but radiology had delivered the results of the test to him. Andrea answered the phone and as she listened to the doctor, she began writing on a piece of paper, 'they found a mass'. At that point, her eyes filled with terror and tears, and she handed me the phone without speaking. She sat back down and began to cradle Ryan in her arms as tears flooded her eyes. I talked to the doctor and he told me that he was consulting with Arkansas Children's Hospital (ACH) about treatment. He told me he would let me know what they said."

My head began to spin and my stomach felt uneasy. I sat back in my chair. As the information had become increasingly intense, I had unconsciously slid to the front of my chair. Quite literally, I was on the edge of my seat with anticipation. Once I had re-seated myself, I asked, "Then what happened?"

Sounding as if he had tried to distance himself emotionally from the events, Chris continued in a droning cadence. "After a few minutes the doctor called back and said ACH wanted Ryan in Little Rock, as soon as possible. He also told me that he had given the nurse an order for Ryan to be given pain medication. They transported Ryan from the waiting area to the emergency room and put an IV in his arm. They gave him the pain medication through the IV. While they were working on inserting the IV, the doctor left his office and drove to the hospital with the CT scan results."

Chris' encounter with the doctor had been disturbing. He explained that the doctor had held the CT scan up to the light and pointed to a large spot on the scan. "I realize you probably don't understand what you are looking at, Mr. Mondy, but I can assure you of one thing. That large spot you see is not supposed to be there."

Sadly, Chris did see the spot. He did not understand what should have been present in a CT scan, but he clearly saw the massive image the doctor had indicated.

Unsure of what to do next, Chris asked the doctor what the next step was. The doctor explained that ACH wanted Ryan transported by ambulance to Little Rock. They were concerned about Ryan making the trip without medical supervision.

Hesitantly, I commented, "Mom said they were airlifting him by helicopter."

He tersely retorted, "Let me finish. While we were talking to the doctor, a nurse came in and told us that ACH had called back and decided that Ryan needed to be in Little Rock quicker than an ambulance could get him there. 'A helicopter will be here within 30 minutes to fly him down to ACH.'"

"Oh, I understand," I meekly added.

"I have to go," Chris snapped. "We are headed home right now pack a bag and pick Ashtyn (their daughter) up from the neighbors."

"Now what?" I wondered. Chris was normally very even-tempered, even under the most difficult of circumstances. The brusqueness with which spoke to me was extremely uncharacteristic and very disconcerting.

I did a quick check and found that it was about four-hundred miles from my house to Little Rock. Home alone and not knowing where else to turn, I sent an e-mail to request prayer support from the members of the church I pastored. I also e-mailed the District Secretary of the Illinois District Church of the Nazarene and asked him to share the prayer request with his entire e-mail contact list.

Laura, my wife, came home and I told her what had happened. She was as shocked as I was to hear the news. I thought about what to do for a few minutes. I did not look forward to a four hundred mile trip that evening, but I thought about the anguish in Chris' voice. I decided that the best solution was to pray about what I should do. I stopped everything and I prayed. Within seconds God impressed upon me that I needed to make the trip to Little Rock.

To say I was a bit unnerved by the conversation with Chris would be an understatement. Darkness had already fallen and I did not wish to begin such a long journey. I wanted to be obedient to what I felt God was directing me to do, so I hesitantly began to pack. While I packed, I kept thinking to myself, "Should I really go?" The answer always came back the same. I needed to be in Little Rock, as soon as possible. Once packed, I loaded my suitcase in the van. I drove to the nearest gas station, filled the van with fuel, and headed south.

Nonna, my mom, Poppa, my dad, and my sister, Jenti, all lived near each other, around Poplar Bluff, Missouri. As I drove south, I called Jenti to find out what her plans were.

"Hello," she muttered between sobs.

"I wondered if you had gone to Little Rock." I said to her.

"No, I was at work when mom and dad left and I couldn't go. Steve doesn't want me driving to Little Rock on my own," she sputtered.

"I will be through Poplar Bluff in one hour. If you want to go to Little Rock, be ready to go and I will stop to get you."

"Let me talk to Steve and I will get back with you." Her voice brightened. She hung up the phone and called Steve, her husband, at work.

In just a few minutes, she called me back brimming with excitement. "Steve said I could go. I called Shannon and she wants to go too, if you have enough room."

Shannon was a cousin who lived near Poplar Bluff.

"Tell Shannon I don't mind if she goes, but she has to be at your house and be ready to go when I get there."

I stopped around the corner from Jenti's house and filled the van up with gas once again. I hopped back in the van and, right on schedule, I rolled into Jenti's driveway. I rushed into her house to use the restroom while they loaded their gear in the van and within ten minutes, we were once again on the road headed toward Little Rock.

As the clock neared 12:30 a.m. on November 4, we pulled into the ACH parking lot. Poppa and Chris were crossing the lot as we arrived. They had gotten something from Chris' van and they were on their way back to Ryan's room. When they saw us, they stopped and waited for us to park. It was easy finding a parking place that late at night, so I quickly parked and we all bounded out of the van. As we approach Chris and Poppa, we inquired about Ryan's status.

"He is resting comfortably right now," Chris replied. He didn't elaborate, but I could tell that he was concerned. He didn't say much, but his body language spoke volumes. He rigidly stood there, with visible tension on his face. Jenti tried to offer a consoling hug, but Chris didn't return the embrace. He had begun the day by going to work about nineteen or twenty hours before. Now he was standing in a hospital parking lot not knowing what the future held for him and his family. He was tired and he was worried. He didn't say a lot, because he did not trust himself to speak without showing some vulnerability.

Chris functioned well under pressure, we both did. However, we had a problem in self-regulation. If we bottled everything inside, we could stay strong and face anything. Chris knew that if he began to let his emotions start to flow, there would not be a way to stop the outpouring. He had gone into defense mode, and the easiest way to keep from saying something he would regret was to say very few words at any one time.

With the realization that we were starting to get cold standing outside, we turned to walk into the building. Chris stepped to the forefront and became the guide leading us to the appropriate entrance. Due to the late hour, only one of the many hospital entrances was utilized. The limited entry point enabled hospital security to be more efficient. Chris spoke at length with security to get each of us a guest pass, which allowed us into the building. After Chris obtained the passes, a guard ushered us to the third floor, where the PICU (Pediatric Intensive Care Unit) was located. As it had only been a few hours since Ryan arrived in the PICU, the staff bent the rules a little to let more than two of us into his room at once. The room was too small for more than three or four visitors, so we took turns going to see Ryan that night.

To say that I received a shock by what I saw when I entered his room would be an understatement. I walked into this tiny room, barely large enough for the hospital bed that Ryan occupied, crowded with family and staff. I looked around the room, which didn't take but a few seconds. The room consisted of a small built-in couch for one person to sleep on, a sink, and a few shelves. Obviously, the room's existence did not merit a need for comfort or for extravagance. When I stepped into Ryan's room, he was watching a movie.

"Well, hello, Uncle Tim. What are you doing here?" he quietly chirped. For a child who had been airlifted to the hospital, he seemed rather exuberant.

I explained I had heard that he was sick so I had come to see how he was doing.

"I got to fly in a helicopter," he bragged, his face glowed with excitement.

"You did?" I answered in mock surprise. I was well aware of the flight.

Ryan furrowed his little brow as he continued, "Yep, but they wouldn't land at McDonalds to get me something to eat."

I did my best to stifle a snicker.

"Well, how are they treating you here at the hospital?" I half-heartedly asked.

"They are really nice," he told me. "They give me all the Sprite that I want, all I have to do is ask for it."

That was a treat for him. His parents didn't let their kids have a lot of soda, so Ryan was impressed that he could have a soda, especially that late at night.

Nurse Valerie stepped up to his bedside and asked Ryan if he needed anything. It was obvious that Ryan had fallen for Nurse Valerie. Anything he wanted, she was right there to make sure he had it. She treated Ryan as if he were royalty.

Someone made a funny remark and everyone in the room started to laugh. Ryan winced in pain and asked us to be quieter.

"I have a headache, can you please quiet down?" he requested as he moved his hands over his ears.

I saw that an IV was in Ryan's arm, but as I looked around, there were no other signs of him being ill. The way he acted when we arrived at the hospital made it seem as if the severity of his condition had been dramatically overstated. Once again, I wondered if I had made a mistake traveling to Little Rock.

We spent a little bit of time in Ryan's room and then one by one we headed to the PICU waiting area. I looked around and saw a whole host of people who were there to check on Ryan. Jenti, Shannon, and I were there. Nonna and Poppa were there. Chris, Andrea, and Ashtyn were there. Additionally, Mames, Randy, and Judy were all present. Randy and Judy had been close friends of Andrea's family for many years. Their daughter, Mames, had been one of Andrea's best friends for years. Randy, Judy, and Mames all lived much closer to ACH than Chris and Andrea did. Andrea had called Randy and Judy to alert them of the situation and ask if they could meet the helicopter when it reached the hospital. They had agreed and then called Mames to tell her the situation. They had all arrived at the hospital about the time the helicopter landed and they had remained throughout the evening.

The clock approached 1:30 a.m. on Saturday morning, and we were all tired. We discussed the situation and decided that we should get two motel rooms for the night. We checked with the receptionist at the desk in the PICU area to find out about nearby accommodations. We asked if any local motels offered special rates for families of ACH patients. We received a list of nearby motels with discounts, but we told the receptionist that we wanted the one that was closest and least expensive. We got the name and directions to that motel and everyone, except for Andrea and Ryan, loaded in the cars and headed to the motel.

Chris' company had an agreement with this motel chain, so he wanted to put the rooms on his account. Since we did not know how long we would need to stay in the motel, he wanted to get the lowest rate possible. Finally, just past 2:00 a.m., we had settled into our rooms. After helping us carry our luggage into the motel, Chris headed back to the hospital. We told him that we would be praying for Ryan and that we would see him about 9:00 a.m., after visiting hours started. The receptionist had informed us that the hours would be much more inflexible when we returned to the hospital because they knew that everyone had made it to the hospital to see Ryan.

After a restless five or so hours of sleep, Nonna called Chris to see how things were going.

"Terrible," Chris responded. "Shortly after I got back last night, Ryan started screaming in agony from the pain. They gave him all of the pain medication that they could give him and when he just kept screaming, they sedated him to let him get some rest."

Hearing the desperation in Chris' voice, Nonna pushed to get everyone ready as quickly as possible, so we could get back to the hospital. The time was just past 8:30 a.m. when we arrived, and visiting hours had not begun. Not knowing whether or not we could gain early admittance, we attempted to open the front door. The door was unlocked, and our entry was gained.

I had been so tired the previous night that I had not paid much attention to the details of our surroundings. Though my sleep had been sparse, I was more alert when we entered this time and I began to absorb more of the environment. As we entered the hospital, I immediately became aware that this place had been created with children in mind.

A massive play area lay off to one side of the entrance. The area had been built partly inside and partly outside of the building. Between the play area and the entrance, a water feature had been built to replicate a serene babbling brook. As the water gurgled and bubbled along its path, it was a calming presence in an otherwise chaotic scene.

After entering the front doors, we walked directly ahead, toward the red elevators. There were two red elevators and to get to the PICU area, we had to take one of the red elevators to the third floor. The elevators in the hospital were color-coded. Any time we asked for directions, the color of the elevator to use would be part of the directions. The red elevators were closest to the front entrance; the green elevators were closer to the emergency entrance, and so on.

The red elevators were the most decorative set in the hospital. They had glass panels on one side so we could view the surroundings as we were shuttled from floor to floor. The layout of the building included a large open shaft approximately sixty feet across, which ran parallel to the sides of the elevator shafts. The shaft started on the ground floor and continued upward for several floors. Three-dimensional artwork was suspended at varying heights in the shaft. As we were transported by the elevator, the artwork could be seen from multiple vantage points.

We rode the elevator to the third floor and when we stepped out of it, we were bombarded with a brightly colored visual sensation. The walls of the hallway we traversed were covered with a beautiful mural. Upon closer inspection of the painting, I determined that it had multiple three-dimensional components included.

One especially interesting aspect of the artwork was the aquarium, which had been built into the wall. Several brightly colored fish swam in the aquarium. The genius of the mural lay in the fact that the overall theme was a stream scene. The aquarium gave us the impression we were looking under the surface of the water. While live fish swam below the surface, images of children had been painted above the surface. The children were involved in activities such as canoeing and lying along the shore reading. As we walked down the hall, we studied the mural. Suddenly, the realization hit us that we were barred from entering the PICU waiting room by a massive set of wooden doors. We did not know how to get beyond the doors. As we discussed the situation, someone walked past us and hit a large button on the wall.

The doors swung open, almost as if someone had uttered those famous words, "Open Sesame."

With the doors open, we continued down the hardwood hallway toward our destination. The deathly silence that enveloped us was interrupted only by the determined footsteps of our tormented little band. The closer we came to the PICU, the more pungent the aroma of disinfectant became.

The PICU layout was similar to many other ICU's that I had visited through the years in checking on my congregants. One corridor led from the elevator toward the PICU. The PICU reception desk was a short way down that hall. At the reception desk, the hall split, forming a T-shape. One short hallway went left into the PICU waiting room and the other hall went to the PICU area. To get into the waiting room, or into the PICU, we had to walk past the reception desk, where a receptionist was on duty twenty-four hours a day.

The receptionist was kept abreast of what was happening in the PICU. One of the duties of the person at the desk was to be an intermediate between the PICU and the waiting room. When we arrived, we explained that we were family members of Ryan Mondy. The receptionist was well of aware of the difficult night Ryan had experienced, so we were allowed into the PICU waiting area. We were not permitted to enter the PICU area though, because visiting hours had not begun.

To gain access to the PICU required going past the receptionist, down the other hallway composing the T-shaped corridor. At the end of the other hall, the PICU opened into a massive hive of activity. There was a central desk area for all of the doctors, nurses, and technicians to work. The desks faced the patient rooms, which had walls made of clear glass, for visibility. This enabled the staff to sit at the desks maintaining the patient charts and still be able to see if their patients were in need of anything. There was somewhere around twenty-five units in the PICU.

After allowing us to enter the PICU waiting room, the receptionist notified Chris we had arrived. A few minutes later, a haggard looking Chris dragged himself to the PICU waiting room and morosely shared Ryan's status. From the 7:00 a.m. phone call until we arrived at the hospital, Ryan's condition had deteriorated. Ryan had started "posturing."

Chris explained "posturing" to us. "The doctor said that there is a fluid build-up inside Ryan's head and his brain is swelling. That is what is causing his headache. The swelling and fluid are putting pressure on his spinal column, causing his extremities to move involuntarily. He is lying there, sedated, and his arms and legs are moving without him doing it. They are concerned that his brainstem is being damaged. If that happens, he can become paralyzed, or worse."

We talked for a few more minutes about Ryan's condition, and then Chris and I left the waiting room and went to Ryan's room. Andrea had remained in the room with Ryan while Chris had trekked to the waiting room to inform us of Ryan's current condition. When we returned to the room, Andrea left so she could join the rest of the family in the waiting room.

When I got to the room, Ryan was on more monitors and IVs than I remembered from the previous night. Chris looked exhausted. That five or so hours of sleep that we had gotten had eluded him due to Ryan's screaming through most of those hours. As we stood in Ryan's room just looking down at his little body, Chris started to open up to me a little bit about what he had heard from the doctors and nurses.

"When we came in yesterday, the doctors were talking about getting an MRI of Ryan's head on Monday. They didn't think they could get him squeezed in for the procedure over the weekend. They told me a little while ago that they were probably going to go ahead and get that MRI today."

I questioned Chris, "Why do they need an MRI, can't they use the CT scan?"

"The CT scan done yesterday only gave them a rough estimate of what they were facing. The MRI will give a more detailed picture of the mass. Once they have a better idea of what they are confronted with, they will have a better idea of how to treat it," Chris countered.

As we stood talking, a nurse came in and told us they going to intubate Ryan, which meant they were going to put a tube down his throat and place him on a ventilator. With the medication, they were giving him to sedate him and the pressure on his brain, his body was having trouble keeping up with breathing.

All of my wonder about whether or not I should have made the trip was gone at this point. Ryan's behavior the night before had only been the calm before the storm.

"After we finish intubating him, the doctor has decided to place a drain in Ryan's skull to try to pull some of the excess fluid out of there," the nurse explained to us. "The cranial pressure is critical as the posturing indicates, but, another complication has shown up. Ryan's pupils are starting to dilate unevenly, which indicates that one side of his brain is affected and the other side is not. I hate to say this, but his pupils are also fixed, they do not react to light any longer."

Fixed pupils were a very bad sign. When the pupils became fixed, it indicated Ryan's brain function had become impaired by the pressure. I hurried back to the waiting room to let Andrea know they were preparing to intubate Ryan. When she heard about the intubation and the drain insertion, she leapt to her feet and raced back to Ryan's room.

Though the rules said only two visitors at a time were allowed in the PICU, I felt I needed to be with Chris and Andrea for moral support. I determinedly stepped to the receptionist desk and proceeded, "I am a minister, as well as Chris' brother. The nurse said they are in the process of intubating Ryan. Is there any way I can be allowed to be back in the unit with Chris and Andrea to offer them some comfort?"

The receptionist allowed me to go back into the unit. Apparently, the person working the reception desk passed the word that I was a preacher, because the rest of the reception staff allowed me a lot of latitude in going to Ryan's room when there were already two people in there. We were always considerate of the other patients and we stayed out of the way when members of the staff were attending to Ryan.

As I approached Ryan's room, Chris and Andrea were standing outside the room looking shell-shocked. Before the intubation procedure began, one of the doctors made Chris and Andrea leave the room. Apparently, he had not been concerned about sounding polite. We watched through the glass walls as the two procedures were simultaneously performed. One group worked on intubating Ryan and the other group began inserting the drain. Medical staff surrounded Ryan's bed. Doctors, technicians, and nurses all moved with amazing speed.

I walked up, put my arms around Chris and Andrea, and told them I wanted to pray with them. As they prayed silently, I prayed aloud, "Our most precious, Heavenly Father, we come to You now on behalf of Ryan. Father, he is in trouble and we are helpless to do anything about it. We know that with You, all things are possible. Please protect this precious child, and please give these doctors the wisdom to care for him. We place all of our trust in You and we are asking that You strengthen and encourage Chris and Andrea as they wait…," I began and I continued the prayer until I ran out of words. When I finished praying, we turned to watch the doctors work on Ryan.

With the procedures completed, one of the doctors came out and apologized for being rude in telling Chris and Andrea to leave the room. Chris assured the doctor that the encounter was not a problem.

Chris looked the doctor in the eye and said with utmost sincerity and determination, "I know you are trying to save my son's life. Nobody in our family will give you any lip and when you tell us to move, we will move. You save my son; we will stay out of your way."

"I appreciate your understanding, Mr. Mondy," the doctor responded. "Ryan's condition has taken a serious turn for the worse. We have decided to perform an MRI as quickly as we can get Ryan prepared. Depending on the results of the MRI, we may have to perform the evacuation today as well."

"Evacuation?" Chris questioned the doctor.

"That is the technical term for removing the mass. Depending on what the MRI shows, we may have to perform surgery today to evacuate, remove, the mass," the doctor compassionately explained.

Less than twelve hours before, Ryan was awake and alert, watching TV and drinking Sprite. Now, he had a drain in his head, an MRI was scheduled and emergency surgery was a strong possibility. Then things turned yet again.

I went back around to the waiting room to let everyone know what had transpired. After I briefed my family, I went back to Ryan's room to be with Chris and Andrea.

When I got back to Ryan's bedside, Chris explained what he had found out about the drain.

"In addition to draining fluid out of Ryan's head, the drain, known as an EVD by the way, is allowing them to monitor the actual pressure in his head. The pressure is too high and they said that the EVD should cause an almost instantaneous drop in the pressure. It hasn't dropped though."

As we stood there discussing the drain and pressure, one of the doctors came up to us to tell us what was going to happen.

The doctor began, "The drain is not causing the decrease in pressure that we had hoped. We only have one course of treatment that we feel we can pursue. We are going to take your son to have an in-depth MRI performed, on the way to the operating room. As quickly as we have the results of the MRI, we will use them to perform the evacuation of the mass."

At approximately 11:00 a.m., we watched as they wheeled Ryan's bed away toward the elevator as they took him to the MRI lab. As the elevator doors closed, a thousand thoughts were flying around inside of my head. The two thoughts that really stuck with me were, "Will I ever see Ryan again?" and "Lord, I don't know why this is happening, but I know that You are in control." One cannot conceive of all the possible questions that come to mind as you watch a six-year-old child go into an elevator with tubes, IVs, ventilator, and a myriad of staff all in tow.

Chris, Andrea, and I began the trek back to the waiting room to let everyone know the new timeline. Everything had happened so quickly. In less than 24 hours, Ryan had gone from a little boy with a headache, to a little boy with a mass in his head causing the headache, to a little boy with a mass in his head causing a headache who was on the verge of brain damage or possibly even death.

As we sat in the waiting room, I talked with Chris and Andrea about creating a CaringBridge website about Ryan. I had become acquainted with CaringBridge through an automobile accident involving a young woman in our community. The young woman, Jaylyn, had been in the hospital for several weeks. Jaylyn's family had created a CaringBridge site to keep any interested persons up to date with information about her condition. I told them that it was nice to be able to read information firsthand from the website. I explained that when I read information from her website, I knew that it was not exaggerated or incorrect. Chris and Andrea were all for setting up a CaringBridge website for Ryan, and since there was a computer in the waiting room for the PICU, I set about creating the website.

There were multiple components to a CaringBridge site. One portion of the site was the journal. In the journal, we were frequently able to add current information about Ryan's condition. Anyone who wanted to read about Ryan's condition could check the journal entries to see what information we had posted. Another vital part of the site was the guestbook. In the guestbook, visitors to the website could post words of encouragement.

At the time I created the site and posted the initial information, Ryan had been gone from us for almost two hours. During the site set-up process, the CaringBridge site generated an e-mail form letter. The letter contained a hyperlink to Ryan's website. Once the site was completed, I sent the e-mail to everyone on my mailing list, including my denomination's District Secretary and asked that everyone who received the e-mail pass it along with a request for prayer. As we received phone calls throughout the afternoon, we shared the information about the website. We continued to ask everyone we encountered to pray for Ryan and visit the website to let us know they were praying for him. We requested that the link and the prayer request be shared with as many people as possible.

While we continued to wait, Chris and Andrea shared more of the details about Ryan's trip from Rogers to Little Rock. Ryan had told us that he had wanted to land at McDonalds to get something to eat; however, there was more to that story. When they would not land, Ryan had asked the crew if they had any food on board the helicopter. If they could not land, he wanted them at least to feed him a snack. The crew explained that there was no food on the helicopter. Ryan promptly told them that if they had allowed his mom on the flight she would have had a snack for him.

About 4:00 p.m., we received a brief update that the surgery was going well and Ryan's vital signs were holding steady. I quickly updated the journal with the information that the surgery continued and all was still going well. In the interim between the creation of the journal and the 4:00 p.m. update, the guestbook had entries from seven different people in four separate states. I called Chris to the computer and showed him the website. He read the guestbook and his eyes began to glisten a little. Chris never publically broke down and wept, he was too macho for such emotion, but there were numerous occasions when his eyes would begin to glisten and tears would form in the corners of his eyes. This was one of those times. The realization that people in other states were concerned about and praying for Ryan touched Chris deeply.

The afternoon trudged on into the evening. Most people in our little band had not eaten properly, some not at all throughout the day. Chris was one of the people who had not eaten and he decided that he wanted a big steak. As we could not get a steak delivered to the hospital, I told him I would go to a restaurant to get one for him. He called Colton's Steakhouse and placed his order. Everyone else decided to have food delivered. While we were getting the order together, a brief update came from the operating room. Ryan's vital signs still looked good and the surgery was still going well.

I took Shannon with me to get Chris' steak. Neither of us was familiar with Little Rock, and since no one really wanted to leave the hospital, I drafted Shannon since she was less surly than Jenti. Emotions were running very high and Shannon had a bit more calm about her than anyone else did, so I drafted her to be my co-pilot. I used an online map service to get directions to the restaurant. We headed out from the hospital, me driving and Shannon reading the directions. All went well until we got close to the restaurant. It was not where it was supposed to be. Shannon read and re-read the directions and then realized that at one point she had misread the decimal point in one of the steps. We were supposed to have gone 0.1 mile not 1.0 miles before we turned.

I became slightly irate with Shannon over the mistake, but then I realized that she had never been to Little Rock either, so I let the error slide. We re-traced our route and still didn't find the restaurant. It was not where the map said it was supposed to be. What had been a mildly irksome moment of Shannon's misreading of the directions suddenly became very disconcerting and quite frustrating. We had been gone from the hospital far longer than I had intended and I was anxious to get back.

Shannon sensed my frustration and she blurted out, "Jesus, please just help us find the restaurant so we can get Chris' food and get back to the hospital." The words had barely cleared her mouth when Shannon squealed with delight, "There it is!"

We had driven past the place three times, but another business obstructed our view of Colton's Steakhouse. God had answered Shannon's prayer and showed us our destination. Without further interruption, we picked up Chris' dinner and headed back to the hospital.

While we were gone, Ryan's surgery was completed and during our absence from the hospital, the neurosurgeon had spoken with Chris and Andrea about Ryan's condition. After Chris and Andrea had spoken with the surgeon, they had gone to Ryan's room to see him. He was in a different room than he was in prior to the surgery. The staff had been very busy getting Ryan settled into his new room, along with all of his monitors and IVs, so they would only allow the parents in the room at that time.

As Shannon and I arrived back at the hospital with Chris' food, we returned to the waiting room to find that the order with everyone else's food had just arrived also. We gathered in a conference room to eat that night, and while we ate, Chris brought us up to speed on all that had transpired while we were getting dinner together.

He began by telling us what the neurosurgeon had reported. "The doctor said the surgery went well, but that he only got a portion of the tumor. One of the pieces of equipment they needed was not working, so they couldn't get all of it."

It was during this conversation that the word "tumor" first entered into the discussion. The doctor did not mince words. He told Chris and Andrea that the tumor was cancerous. According to the doctor, he had removed a "bloody glia tumor" with "fingers" which had intertwined themselves with the nerves in Ryan's brain. At that time, he warned Chris and Andrea that a second surgery might be necessary to remove the rest of the tumor, on a day when the equipment was functioning.

Chris told us that the doctor had looked at him and said, "Mr. Mondy, today we saved your son's life, if we have to go back in to get the rest we will deal with that at a later time."

When we heard the doctor's report, we were a little more relieved. To us, it seemed that the doctor was assuring us Ryan had survived the surgery. In effect, I guess that was what he said. However, we extrapolated a little much and assumed that with his comments he meant that everything was going to be fine. He had not meant to give us false hope; he was trying to let us know Ryan had survived that far into the day. Everything else we only assumed, the doctor had not told us that Ryan was fine. We were a bit downcast at the same time, because we now knew that Ryan had cancer and that scared us.

Struggling through weariness to remember all that the surgeon had said, Chris continued to share with us. "The surgeon told us he had done his best to minimize the nerve damage. He said the location of the tumor would most likely cause problems with Ryan's left side. The tumor had intertwined itself around the nerves, so he removed as much of the tumor as he could without bothering the nerves. We were warned there would probably be some loss of movement in Ryan's left arm and leg." Chris' face distorted slightly as he remembered the most painful portion. "The surgeon told us there was a chance that Ryan could be completely paralyzed on the left side. They will not know the extent of nerve damage until Ryan is awake."

Following the consultation with the surgeon, the nurses allowed Chris and Andrea to go into the room with Ryan for a bit. Andrea had stayed in the room while Chris had returned to eat his dinner and share the doctor's report with us.

"How was Ryan when you went into his room?" Nonna queried.

Chris choked up a bit at this point as he continued, "I asked Ryan if he could hear me. He had that tube down his throat, so I told him that if he could hear me to open his eyes big and wide. He opened them all the way. I asked him if he could move his fingers and toes and he tried to move them. He even moved his left leg a little bit, so I know he is not completely paralyzed."

Chris had gone on to converse with Ryan for a few more minutes before he came to join us for dinner. He had Ryan open his eyes wide for yes and close his eyes if the answer to a question was no. It seemed to work pretty well, but as the doctors had ordered heavy doses of painkillers for him, Ryan had drifted in and out of consciousness frequently. Chris had decided to let Ryan rest and get something to eat for himself.

While we were eating, one of the nurses came and told us they had finished settling Ryan into his room. She said that even though it was past visiting hours, we could go in and see him before we left the hospital. As I was finished eating, I went to Ryan's room to check on him. The image of him lying in the bed, attached to all of the tubes and monitors, instantly etched itself into my mind forever.

His face was battered, swollen, and bruised. Surgical gauze encased his tiny head, as if he were some form of Egyptian mummy. The vast number of IV lines criss-crossing one another looked like some form of sterile snake pit. At that time there were eighteen different IV lines connecting the IV pumps to Ryan's body. Ryan lay deathly still as I entered the room, sedated to remove him from the world of pain in which his body was entrenched. Sterile tape covered the intubation tube to hold it in place, the ventilator continued to breathe for Ryan.

I peered more closely at the IV lines. Each was labeled with the type of medicine that was flowing through them into his tiny frame. With my eyes, I traced each of the lines. Some terminated in his feet, some in his hands, and some in his arms. More tape had been applied to hold each of these lines in place.

Ryan lay bare-chested, as they did not want clothing to be in the way when they listened to his heart and lungs. His legs were bare as well. Only a thin blanket gave him some slight measure of modesty. They needed complete access to his body, and they did not know if they would have the luxury of time to move a pants leg or undo a button.

From under the gauze turban, the EVD line snaked its way up an IV pole to a collection vessel. Fluid from inside Ryan's head drained into a vessel, which was marked with graduated increments. The increments measured how many milliliters of fluid drained from his head. As I traced that line, I saw that the collection vessel was distinctly tinged with blood.

Betadine, the disinfectant they used to sterilize his skin before making an incision, stained his forehead. The brown solution extended well below the bottom of the surgical dressing.

An oxygen sensor was on one finger, and a blood pressure cuff was on his arm. Additionally, he was connected to a heart monitor so they could keep track of his pulse rate. The monitors told me that he was still alive; however, his ashen complexion and lifeless form tried to convince my mind otherwise.

All I could do was slink back to the room where everyone else awaited a turn to visit his room. I tried to warn everyone about the scene one would witness when entering Ryan's room; however, the grim reality of his condition made my attempt to describe the scene rather futile. One by one, individuals went to see him. Utter dismay clouded the faces of those returning from Ryan's room. More than a few tears fell that night.

Ryan was out of surgery and back in PICU and it was time for us to leave. Every one of us was emotionally drained and exhausted. It was not something we necessarily wanted to do, but all of us except for Chris and Andrea left the hospital and headed back to the motel for the night. We returned to the motel to spend yet another fitful night trying vainly to get the rest we all so desperately needed.

Sunday morning dawned with a sense of foreboding spreading across each of us. Awakening in the motel, we all realized that the events, which had taken place, were not all part of some bad dream. It was all real, too real in fact.

We called the hospital and talked with Chris. He said he had not slept much as he was in the room with Ryan. He said that the warning sirens on the monitors had frequently sounded throughout the night. Andrea had slept in the waiting area, as there was only room for one of them in Ryan's room.

Ryan had made it through the night, which was a blessing to hear. We dressed and went to the hospital. We got to the PICU waiting room right about 9:00 a.m., almost twelve hours after the completion of the surgery. Chris was in the waiting room when we arrived.

Poppa ventured to ask the question that we all were wondering, "So, how is the little man this morning?"

"Well, he made it through the night," Chris responded. "They are going to take him down for a CT scan a little later this morning."

I think Sunday, November 5, 2006, was probably one of the most heart-wrenching days of my life.

The ability Ryan had to communicate by opening or closing his eyes immediately after the surgery was very short-lived. During the surgery, an incision which was several inches long had been made in the soft tissue of Ryan's head and then a portion of his skull had been cut away to access the tumor. Following the evacuation procedure, the skull had to be reconstructed. Once the skull fragments were repositioned, they had to be secured in place with tiny screws. Once the skull was secured, the incision was sutured shut. The pain associated with that type of procedure and the subsequent post-operative swelling caused the doctors to order continued sedation for Ryan. In their opinion, pain medication would have been inadequate to alleviate all of the pain.

The surgeon had removed a portion of the tumor, a portion nearly two inches square. The hope was that it would relieve the pressure in Ryan's head. However, following the surgery, fluid began to fill the void left by the tumor removal. Post-operative swelling also contributed to the complications in trying to regulate the deadly pressure in Ryan's head. The doctors told us that from a neurological standpoint, the pressure caused by the fluid in Ryan's head was nearly as dangerous as the pressure previously caused by the tumor. The management of that fluid pressure became a crisis, which would be ongoing for an excruciatingly long time.

I began to roam the halls of the hospital while I waited. I went downstairs to the computer lab that the hospital had on the first floor. I decided to search on the internet and see what information I could find about a glia tumor. I Googled "glia tumor" and several hundred thousand matches were returned. I tried to wade through some of the articles but as I read, I became overwhelmed with information. I decided to stop researching the topic. I had not realized how many different types of cancer there were. Not just cancer, but also more specifically, types of brain cancer. As I looked at the information I found, it ran the gamut from moderate concern to impending doom. There were different forms of cancer and for each form of cancer, there were different levels, stages, or categories. Some forms of cancer were operable while others were not. Some used chemotherapy, some used radiation, and some both. The outlook for some forms of cancer was positive; however, the prognosis was rather depressing for other forms. I ran across one that said there was only an eleven percent likelihood of a patient surviving more than two years. Another said there was a high level of recovery.

Cancer is a broad topic to research. I began to understand why the doctors did not postulate a course of treatment following the surgery. The doctor had told Chris and Andrea, they would not address the treatment of the remaining tumor until after they had received the pathology report back, which would take about ten business days. The pathology results were extremely important in determining a course of treatment; therefore, they wanted to be one-hundred percent certain about the form and stage. A biopsy of the tumor had been sent to the in-hospital lab and to two external labs for testing. The three labs would report their findings to the doctors, who would compare the results. Once all three reports completely agreed, the doctors would plan a course of treatment. Only after the doctors agreed on a plan of action would the family be told the pathology results. If any of the labs had any differences in their report, they would need to explain the discrepancy. In the end, all three reports would agree. If one lab found something the others did not, they would justify their conclusion. If two found something, the third lab would re-evaluate and see if they had missed something. We would have a unanimous agreement before we moved forward.

I decided to leave the research alone as I was becoming more overwhelmed and more discouraged as I read. I did not think I could bear any more bad news. We did not know yet what type of cancer Ryan had and the prognosis had a whole spectrum of possibilities depending on the type and stage of the cancer. I decided there was no need in becoming more upset, so I left the computer lab and went back to see Ryan for a bit.

When I visited the room again, I realized that the cancer was actually a secondary concern, at least at that point in time. The crisis of the day was the pressure inside of his head. There were two pressure readings that were critical, the ICP or inter-cranial pressure, the pressure inside of his head, and CPP or cranial profusion pressure, the pressure of blood flow inside of his head. The ICP was supposed to be below 20 and the CPP was supposed to be above 60; however, in Ryan's case those numbers would often become reversed. A high ICP could cause death or paralysis. A low CPP could cause brain damage. The pressure combinations that happened were extremely dangerous. In addition, Ryan's heart rate would race at times and his monitors were constantly going off. I watched the monitors fluctuate and listened to the alarms repeatedly sound. When I reached the point I could not handle any more, I left Ryan's room and went back to the waiting room.

During the first part of the morning, Ryan was very heavily sedated and sleeping. Periodically the sedative would start to become insufficient and Ryan would rouse a bit. When he roused from his sedation, he tried to point to his mouth and let the nurse know he was hungry. Sometime during the morning on Sunday, a feeding tube was inserted through Ryan's nose, down the back of his throat and into his stomach. A little before noon, Ryan took a turn for the worse.

To assist in stabilizing the pressure issue, the doctors determined that Ryan needed placed on a cooling blanket. The blanket had fittings that attached to a heat pump. The pump could either heat or cool water. Once the water reached the desired temperature, it flowed through channels contained inside of the blanket. In Ryan's case, the machine chilled the water to a point that caused his body temperature to drop to around 90°F. We had gotten to the hospital around 9:00 a.m., and within three hours, Ryan's condition had gone downhill quickly.

The scenario we experienced seemed very surreal. If a Salvador Dali painting came to life, it would have been something like that day. Nothing made sense. What seemed bad was in fact worse. I had trouble sitting still, so I would wander around the hospital. Typically, when I began to roam the halls, I would end my sojourn at Ryan's bedside. The first time I went in after they placed him on the cooling blanket was horrible.

When they placed Ryan on the cooling blanket, they had to prevent his body from shivering due to the cold. They placed him in a chemically induced coma, which prevented him from any self-induced movement. When I picked up his hand, it had the feel of death: cold and lifeless. As I stood there staring down at that frail little body, tears began to fill my eyes. His face was so swollen from the surgery it looked as if his entire head had ruptured. His right eye was swollen to the point that it appeared as if at any moment it could burst. His entire body was completely lifeless and unbelievably cold. The ventilator continued to breathe for him, and with each artificial breath, his tiny chest would rise and fall. Every measurable vital sign that one can imagine was monitored and recorded. I just stood there looking at him in amazement. I wondered just how much fight this little guy could possibly have in him. As I was standing there, I felt the presence of God enter the room and something deep within spoke to me and told me to pray for Ryan right then.

In the Bible, in the book of James, chapter 5 it says:

> " *[14]Is any one of you sick? He should call the elders of the church to pray over him and anoint him with oil in the name of the Lord. [15]And the prayer offered in faith will make the sick person well; the Lord will raise him up." (NIV, James 5:14-15).*

In an instant, I grasped that lifeless little hand and I began to pray as I had never prayed before. I called upon God to restore this little one's life and to bring about his healing. I claimed the promise of James 5. As my prayer concluded, I sensed that something changed. I had only been in the room for a few minutes, but I could tell that something was different from when I had entered the room. I believe I had an encounter with God Almighty there in Ryan's room. I also believe that things would have turned out very differently had I not been obedient to what I felt led to pray at that instant.

I left the room, went down to the lobby away from all of my family, and called my wife, Laura.

I broke down in tears while I was on the phone with her. "I don't know how much more he can take. He looks so bad. I tried to research the type of tumor the surgeon said he removed and I probably shouldn't have. I feel like I am losing my grip. Everywhere I look, there are sick kids. It is unbearable here. I keep hearing helicopters land, and I know that every time one lands, it is another kid who is really in trouble, otherwise there would be no need to be airlifted. This place, it just wears on you knowing that all of the patients are kids."

Laura did her best to comfort me and by the time I got off the phone, I had emptied myself of despair. It was a very cathartic experience. She shared with me that the congregation had gathered that morning for special prayer for Ryan. She let me know that I was not alone in the prayer battle. I suddenly realized that I was not in control of what happened. I also knew that the doctors were not in charge. I came to realize that Ryan's ability to survive rested in his ability to fight and God's ability to sustain him as he fought.

As early afternoon rolled around, Mames came to the hospital. I overheard her telling Jenti, in hushed tones, about what she had found out from the internet. Mames was extremely upset and Jenti was as well. I am glad that by that time I had experienced both my meltdown and my time of prayer with Ryan. I told them that I had done the same thing and that I had become just as overwhelmed with the information. I encouraged them not to become distraught over what they had learned from the internet because the pathology results were several days away. I reminded them that the prognosis was very different depending on the stage and form of cancer.

"Besides," I said, "There is no need fretting about that right now; they won't do anything about the cancer for at least a month." That piece of information startled them and they asked what I meant. I shared, "In a case like Ryan's, the surgical incision has to heal before any cancer treatment can be done. No chemotherapy or radiation will take place for at least a month, giving the incision time to heal. The nurse told me that while he is healing, the pathology results will be generated. In effect, we won't be waiting on pathology results; we will be waiting for his body to heal from the surgery. The time for pathology overlaps with the time for healing so when the pathology results are ready, the body will also be ready. Thus, there will not be any loss of time because of the lab work." It was all very neatly packaged. I believe that after we talked, the girls felt better. I know I did.

I had only planned to stay in Little Rock a day or two, but the critical nature of Ryan's condition made me realize that I needed to stay so I could support Chris and Andrea any way possible. I called Laura again and talked with her about what I should do in the coming days. She agreed that I should stay in Little Rock and we decided that she would fly to Little Rock and join me as quickly as possible. Unfortunately, she could not get there before Thursday night. At that point, I committed to staying until the next weekend.

Early that evening, I persuaded Chris to leave the hospital for a while. We went out to eat and while we had dinner, I got a chance to talk with Chris about the future.

When I was alone with the nurses, I began to question them about Ryan's prognosis. The nurses had expressed to me that Ryan's mobility was speculative at best, assuming that he lived through the next few days. While we ate, I broke this news to Chris.

"I know, they told me the same thing," he said.

With tears in his eyes, Chris looked at me and said, "I don't care if he is crippled; I just want to take my little boy home again."

At that moment, I knew that no matter what happened Chris was going to be able to step up and carry the burden that was placed on him. He had placed his focus squarely on Ryan. He did not have high and lofty ambitions; he simply wanted to take his son home. I felt that come what may, Chris would be able to work through it. It had been a difficult decision for me to stay in Little Rock. During that conversation, I realized that God had been faithful in helping me make the correct choice. Chris needed my support and I was glad I had stayed so that I could offer it to him.

Chris and I returned to the hospital after our meal. At that time, we still did not have a clear understanding as to the severity of Ryan's condition. If we had known what the coming days held, we would have probably given up hope. God protected us from future knowledge and He was faithful to protect our hearts each step of the journey. It seemed an eternity since I had received the call from Nonna, but in reality, it had been 48 hours. Sadly, the first 48 hours were not the worst to come.

A Week of Horrors

One "bright spot" had occurred just before the paralytic was administered: Ryan had moved his left leg. It had been a slight movement, but a nurse confirmed that the movement was voluntary. Ryan had moved his leg; it had not been a muscle spasm. The movement indicated that Ryan wasn't paralyzed on his left side; however, movement and mobility are two very different topics. One cannot have mobility without movement; however, being able to move a limb does not insure being able to use that limb efficiently. It was not much hope, but at the least, it was more positive than anything else that happened that day.

By Sunday night, the number of entries in the CaringBridge guestbook inspired Chris to set a goal. He decided that he would like to have at least one person from each of the 50 states sign the guestbook and indicate that they would pray for Ryan. Assuming that Ryan would awaken from his chemical coma, Chris desired the opportunity to show Ryan that someone had been praying for him in each state. We found a printable map on the internet and printed it. Chris bought a package of markers and began to color each state as a representative signed the guestbook. In the nightly website update, Chris mentioned his goal and asked website visitors to spread the word about Ryan. Chris started calling his project the "Nation of Prayer Map." The map hung on the wall at all times, unless it was receiving an update. As the shifts changed, word of the map spread throughout the hospital and people began to visit Ryan's room just to see the map. That map became a visual point of inspiration. One glance at the map and we knew we were not in the battle alone. God's children all around the country were joining us as we prayed for Ryan.

Monday morning came after a fitful night of sleep. Jenti had to return home that day. The plan was for her husband, Steve, to travel to Little Rock that morning. He would then return home that afternoon with Jenti and her belongings. That morning, while Steve was en route to Little Rock, we all went to the hospital to await the outcome of another day. We spoke with Chris by phone early that morning, before visiting hours started, to find out how the night had passed. The report we received, before we reached the hospital that morning, was not good.

During the night, the respiratory therapist had determined that Ryan had a build-up in his left lung. The therapist started treatment, utilizing a CPT. The CPT was a massager that pounded lightly on Ryan's chest and sides. The motion of the massager caused the build-up to be broken up and then the loosened matter was suctioned out of his lung via a tube connected to the ventilator. The pressures had not stabilized, and Ryan's overall condition had not improved since we'd left the night before.

When we arrived at the hospital that morning, Chris was a walking zombie. It had been very difficult for Chris to sleep in Ryan's room. When one of Ryan's vital signs exceeded an acceptable level, the alarms on the monitors sounded. The instability of Ryan's body caused this to become a nearly continuous cacophony of warning sirens. Assuming that Chris had dropped off to sleep, the sirens would yank him back into the nightmarish reality that he had briefly tried to escape through sleep. When the frustration level about not being able to sleep became intolerable, Chris would get out of bed and begin to roam the halls and waiting rooms near the PICU. Through the frustration, Chris found a positive way to deal with his inability to sleep. Chris began utilizing those hours to visit CaringBridge websites. Most of the sites he visited linked him to a subsequent site. He would move from site to site, throughout the late night and early morning hours. At each site he visited, he would leave words of encouragement. When I found out what he had been doing, I was very impressed. In the midst of the greatest crisis he had ever faced, Chris was offering words of encouragement to others, many of whom were in similar situations. As a result of Chris' many kind words, numerous people became acquainted with Ryan's website. These people would often reciprocate the kind words and assure Chris and family that they had added Ryan to their prayer lists. This helped to expand the base of people praying which, in turn, helped in the completion of the "Nation of Prayer Map."

Andrea was very quiet during this time. She wandered from Ryan's room to the waiting room then back to Ryan's room. There was a little washer and dryer in the PICU waiting area, so Andrea worked on keeping the few items of clothing they had brought with them clean. I learned just how resourceful Andrea could be during those days in the waiting room. Every time someone would comment about needing something, she said, "I have that" and she would reach inside her jacket and pull it out. At first, I thought she had taken up magic. At one point she reached in and pulled a full size box of tissues out of her pocket, the kind that are in a rectangle box about two inches thick. It was like watching a magician pull a rabbit out of a hat. In would go her empty hand and out would come her hand with whatever someone had asked for, whether it was a snack, medicine, tissue or some other item. Finally, I could not stand it any longer and I made her take the jacket off and let me see the inside of it. The jacket must have been created with either magicians or moms in mind. A second layer of material was sewn inside the jacket, creating massive pockets. I am not sure how she was able to walk around with the extra weight of the stuff in her pockets, but she managed.

By Monday morning, I had lost count of how many people had visited the hospital with care baskets for the family: snacks, toiletries, puzzle books and toys for Ashtyn and Ryan. In addition to caring for the physical needs, some people began caring for the fiscal needs. Collections had been taken at Chris' office and at the school Ryan attended. One of the civic organizations in Pea Ridge, the town in which Chris' family lived, had jumped into the fray and donated money as well. A bank account was opened in Pea Ridge and anyone who wanted to contribute to Ryan's cause could deposit money directly into that account. The level of concern strangers had for our family was extremely humbling. We will never know all of the people who contributed either financially or with gifts of any sort, but rest assured God knows.

A little before noon I went in to see Ryan. I slipped my cell phone out and snapped a quick picture of Ryan. I wanted to be able to remember what he looked like at that point. He actually looked a little better on Monday than he had on Sunday. The fluid, which caused the swelling of his right eye, was apparently moving toward his left eye. I was concerned about that, but the nurse said the fluid would continue to shift as the days passed and gravity caused the fluid to move lower down his face. The swelling would continually relocate until his body could absorb all of the excess fluid. On Monday morning, instead of having one grotesquely swollen eye, Ryan's entire face began to swell.

The fight to keep his body temperature regulated was ongoing. I spoke with the nurse on duty at the time and we had a long talk. "Is he starting to stabilize?" I asked.

"Not really, but he has stopped the massive fluctuations that he was having yesterday. When his pressures do go wacky, he is tolerating the adjustments fairly well."

By adjustments, she meant the different chemicals the nurses were manipulating to gain the desired monitor readings. As one pressure would spike, an adjustment in the amount of one medication was typically required. When a different pressure dropped too low, the nurses would adjust a different medication. The delicate balancing act the nurses were performing allowed Ryan to live. They could not, or would not, guarantee Ryan would come through that time without brain damage. The best they could offer us, at least as far as hope was concerned, was that Ryan was still alive, and that meant he had a chance to recover. When she informed me that he was tolerating the adjustment, that meant his body was reacting positively to the medications.

"So could we say that he is 'critically stable'?" I asked her.

"If it makes you feel better, yes, you could say he is 'critically stable'. Just don't build that term up too much. He is far from completely stable yet."

As we continued to talk, she could tell I was not satisfied with the prognosis, and she did offer one final word of comfort before I left Ryan's room. The nurse told me that if a patient followed the "book" on recovery, after about forty-eight hours post-surgery, the worst should be over and recovery would begin. Unfortunately, in the days to come, we came to understand that Ryan had not studied the "book."

The number of adjustments that were made was amazing. The nurses were charting every vital statistic about Ryan. They had a large chart that contained various readings including blood work results, ICP/CPP pressure readings, heart rate, and blood pressure. Chart entries were included for all adjustments to the medications. This allowed the doctors and nurses to know, at a glance, how to proceed. If the ICP went up, they could look to the chart and see what adjustments to make to bring it down and what adjustments his body would not tolerate at that time. If Ryan's sodium levels were too high on the blood work, extra saline was not an option. If the sodium levels were acceptable, extra saline helped to bring the ICP down. Extra saline was not possible on a continual basis though, because this caused an overall increase in the sodium level that was in Ryan's body. If the nurses left the saline content higher, there was nothing that could be done to adjust the ICP if it elevated. Every measurement was vital and scrupulous care was given to recording this life-saving data.

From my non-medical perspective, it appeared that in the hospital, there is "critical care," and then there is "Critical Care," the latter being those patients in an ICU who are the most at-risk. If that designation might stand up to scrutiny, then I would say that Ryan was in "CRITICAL CARE." The nurse had allowed me to optimistically coin a phrase of 'critically stable' to describe Ryan's status, but we all knew that with one uncontrollable spike, Ryan might be brain damaged, or he could die. The more I spoke with different nurses, the better I understood just how critical Ryan was. Ryan looked bad and the room looked intimidating with all of the monitors, gauges, and pumps. From the discussion with the nursing staff, it appeared that Ryan was even more critical than we had initially been led to believe. Quite literally, Ryan was only minutes from death before the surgery. To our dismay, we continued to find that, for days following the surgery, he was continually only minutes away from death. If one nurse made a mistake, if one doctor made a bad call, if Ryan rejected any of the attempts, if, if, if…the possibilities were utterly endless as to bad things that could happen.

When I had been in the room for as long as I could stand it, I went back to the waiting room. Steve had arrived to pick Jenti up and take her home. Chris and I usually teased Steve relentlessly. We did it because we liked him. In our family, the more we liked someone the more we teased him or her. Steve never knew what to expect from Chris or me. I did not feel up to kidding around at this juncture, so I did not tease him. We had been trying to forewarn everyone about the nightmare they were preparing to enter by going to visit Ryan. We had grown somewhat accustomed to the scene, but first time visitors to the room were always shocked by what they witnessed.

"Steve," I began, "brace yourself before you go into that room. It is very bad. Ryan looks horrible and all of those monitors and sounds will freak you out." I tried to explain what he would witness when he walked into the room. "When you walk in, the first thing you will see is that ghostly pale little body. He can't move and won't know you are even in the room. If you touch his skin, you will think he is dead because he is so cold. They have him paralyzed with medicine to keep his body from shivering. While you stand there looking at him, that chiller will kick on, or the ventilator will gurgle and sputter and those sounds will make you jump. You need to realize that even though he looks like he is breathing, the ventilator is doing that for him."

I continued telling him the horrors of going in to see Ryan for the first time. I wanted him to be aware of the scene. I didn't want him to walk in unprepared and pass out or something, we didn't need that kind of drama added to everything else. "Be prepared for the alarms to go off while your standing in there and step back when you hear them because at least one nurse will come barreling through to get to that alarm. Stay out of their way, or they will run over you."

Steve looked at me and his eyes were wide. He was not sure if I was kidding or not, but when he looked to Jenti, she assured him that I was serious and Ryan really was that bad. Steve looked back to me in wonderment. I could almost tell that his mind was wondering how something like that could be true. Jenti told him she would go with him back to see Ryan, and so around the corner they went.

When they returned from the room, Steve walked in and sat down. He appeared shaken by what he had seen. He looked at me and thanked me for warning him. Even though I had warned him, it had not truly prepared him for what he witnessed when he walked into the unit. I knew the look on his face. I knew the pain in his chest. I knew the instability he was feeling. I knew, because I had been there repeatedly over the past few days.

The room was so cold, partially because of the cooling blanket and partially because the thermostat had been turned down to aid the cooling blanket. Standing in the room without a jacket would almost assuredly cause one to leave the room shivering. The smells of disinfectant were overpowering at times. No flowers were allowed in the room to improve the smell. Germs were not acceptable, and so everyone had to wash with disinfecting soap every time they went into the room. If anyone chose to enter that tomblike cavern, the status of observer was forever lost. To step into that icy, sterile maw of death, was to step into Ryan's world. Standing at the bedside, one could not help but unconsciously begin breathing in synchronization with the ventilator. It was too easy to become lost in time as one stared into that battered, bruised little face. Every visitor would yearn to change places with him. Their hearts would begin to ache, and they could not explain why. Time crept by so slowly that it was hard to notice its passing. Astonishment crept over anyone who entered the room as they became lost in a world of wonderment at how one little boy could undergo so much pain and suffering. A visitor's legs would begin to shake and a shiver would race up the spine, hands would begin to lose all feeling. When no more could be tolerated, the guest would turn to leave the room. As each person emerged from the doorway, we could tell that another life, like each of ours, had been forever altered. He or she had just stepped into a nightmare, yet this one was very real. No Freddy Kruger, no Jason, death was nearby and one could sense that it was trying desperately to step out of the shadows and claim Ryan's life. Unexpectedly, stepping out of the room caused remorse to try to grip each person who had entered the room. It felt as if guilt would rip the beating heart from its home in the chest of the one who had escaped the nightmare. It was nearly impossible not to feel guilty, for everyone that entered Ryan's world was allowed to leave, except for Ryan. Ryan was trapped in that horror and no one knew if he would ever escape.

It took Steve a little while to recover from what he had witnessed. He sat and talked for a while longer and then it was time for him and Jenti to leave. I know that it was extremely difficult for them to leave, but Jenti had to get home so she could go to work on Tuesday and so did Steve.

Shortly after Steve and Jenti left, we found out that the doctor had ordered another MRI. This was not good news. Much of the equipment that was attached to Ryan was not compatible with the MRI machine. All of the electric pumps that controlled his medicine flows had to be changed to manual pumps, and with the numerous pumps that were connected to Ryan that took a long time.

As we expected, it took more time for Ryan to get ready than to actually get his MRI. We anxiously awaited his return to his room. There was nothing we could do, not even stand by his bedside during his absence. He was gone and we did not know when he would be back. We also knew that while he was in his bed and the nurse was right by his side he was in critical condition. We had no idea how his little body would respond to the trauma of being unhooked from some of the machines and being moved through the hospital. We did not know if he was still on the chilling blanket. We did not know how his body temperature was doing. Most importantly, we did not know how those all-important pressures were doing. The time he was gone for the MRI was a very tense time. The concern, due to all of the uncertainty, was palpable. We breathed a collective sigh of relief when we learned that the MRI was over and that Ryan was back in his room.

The attending physician spoke with Chris after Ryan was back from the MRI. The doctor told Chris that if the pressures did not stabilize very quickly, they would need to do another procedure to insert a second drain inside of Ryan's head. The doctors were concerned that the constant stress on Ryan's other organs, due to the constant rising and lowering of the pressure inside of Ryan's head, could cause more complications. They could not predict what would happen if they continued to work, solely on regulating the pressures and letting Ryan's body try to recover at its own pace. We had wondered about those ourselves, so it did not come as a surprise when the doctor broached the topic. We had seen Ryan's heart rate skyrocket when his pressures would change. We had also witnessed his blood pressure go from being very high to very low, all depending on what medications were administered to regulate either the ICP or the CPP or both. The only two options that remained were Ryan stabilizing on his own, or inserting the second drain.

The stresses of the MRI had not pushed Ryan over the edge. He had made it to the testing area, had the MRI, and made it back to his room. When Ryan returned, the nurses had to go through the process of reconnecting all of the electric pumps. I asked one of the nurses why they bothered switching all of the pumps back to the electric pumps. She explained, "We would rather not have to, but those MRI compatible pumps were very expensive and the hospital only has a limited number of them. Every time we have a PICU patient that needs an MRI, we have to go through this process. We have to switch them out one pump at a time and keep all of the lines straight."

It was a lengthy, tedious process of tracing each line from the pump to where it entered into Ryan's body, but it was essential to ensure that the correct line correlated with the correct pump. Some of the medications interacted with each other if they came into direct contact with one another. If the incompatible medicines pumped through the same line, solids would precipitate out of the liquids and block the line. The nurses were not thrilled about the doctor ordering the MRI, because they knew how much difficulty was involved in prepping Ryan for the MRI. They also realized that if the doctor ordered the MRI, there was a genuine need for the test.

Following the procedure and subsequent conversations with the doctor and nurses, we figured out there were two reasons for the MRI. Initially, the doctors wanted to see how Ryan's brain was responding to the surgery, evaluating the swelling and fluid level. The second reason, according to the doctor's conversation with Chris, was related to the possibility of the second drain. The doctor said if they needed to place the second drain that Ryan's brain was so malformed due to swelling they required an MRI to know the precise location the drain would be most productive. If a second drain were added, the procedure would not be as simple as the placement of the first drain. The second drain, if added, would require one end of a tube being inserted into Ryan's stomach and the other inserted into his head. This would all be under the skin. They would make an incision in Ryan's head, snake the drain line down through his body into his stomach and then insert the other end into his brain. The surgeon informed Chris that it would be a permanent drain. It would continually remove excess fluid out of Ryan's head and transfer it into his stomach, where the body would absorb the fluid back into his system.

Shortly after Ryan returned to his room, visiting hours ended. Nonna, Poppa, Ashtyn, and I had to leave the hospital. Chris checked the guestbook before we left the hospital and it offered us a ray of hope on an otherwise dismally clouded day. The online plea for prayer support was being answered and prayer warriors were springing up all across the country.

Chris whipped out his handy pack of markers and began to color each new state that was represented. He took a pen and wrote Iraqi out in the Atlantic Ocean. On top of the crisis with Ryan, Andrea's brother, Steve, had recently been deployed to Iraqi. When he found out about Ryan, he visited the website and let us know he was praying for Ryan.

When Chris finished coloring, I asked, "So how many states are we up to?"

"Twenty-three," he responded. "Almost half the nation is praying for Ryan."

We were tired, but we did not want to leave. If we had not been directed to leave, we might have stayed later, but as it were, we were ushered out of the waiting room. The cleaning crew came in to tidy the place up after visiting hours each night. They wouldn't interrupt the families during visiting hours, but when it was time for us to go, it was time for them to get started and they were anxious to get to work. The visiting hours had been relaxed for us over the weekend, but we quickly found out that weeknights were a lot different. When weeknight visiting hours were over, we were expected to be gone. They really didn't like us waiting until 9:00 p.m. to leave; it was desirable for us to be out of the building by the time visiting hours ended. So much so that at 9:00 p.m. sharp, the front doors to the hospital were locked and we had to walk around the building to get to our car. We didn't realize that on Monday night, so we left a few minutes after 9:00 and ended up walking around the building. We went back to the motel that Monday night and we knew that Ryan had two very different possibilities for the coming day. If, as the nurse had suggested, the most critical time had passed, Ryan would start getting better soon. However, it was a distinct possibility that the doctors would order the insertion of the second drain. We didn't know what the next day would hold, but we knew that Ryan was not doing well. He had survived a full forty-eight hours following the operation and that was a good sign. As I lay in my bed at the motel, I prayed until I couldn't stay awake any longer. I fell asleep praying for God to continue sustaining our family as we went through the ordeal and I prayed that God would give Ryan the strength to be able to fight through this time, and then I slept.

Tuesday morning dawned and we arose after a decent night's sleep. As we talked about the new day, we were cautiously optimistic. Ryan had made it through the worst day, at least according to the "book." We hoped and we prayed that today would be the start of Ryan's road to recovery. Nonna spoke with Chris on the phone before we went to the hospital. Chris informed Nonna that Ryan had gone through the night much as he had faced the previous nights and days. Stability had not miraculously arrived overnight. As we drove to the hospital, our optimism had begun to wane. The information from Chris had indicated that it would be another very long day of peaks and valleys.

I walked into Ryan's room when we arrived at the hospital and the place had begun to look like a zoo. The rules prohibited Ryan from having any flowers, but he could have stuffed animals and balloons. The nurses encouraged us to share that information with everyone who wondered what they could do to help. The nurses told us that they would use stuffed animals to prop up Ryan's arms and legs. To keep circulation going as it should be, the nurses routinely moved Ryan's extremities. Sometimes they would need to lower one arm and raise the other and when that happened, they would use a little animal to support the arm that needed a lower elevation and a larger animal to raise the elevation of the other. We had communicated that information on the website and within hours, the room began to fill with animals and balloons. The nurses had said they liked the critical cases to have balloons so that when the patients' eyes were open, they could see the bright and cheerful balloons floating in the air. It kept the patients from having to strain their necks to see their surroundings. Balloons allowed the patients to lie on their backs and see something other than ceiling tiles.

The nurses kept talking about the "book" on patient recovery. We were told that if things went by the "book," a patient would be better after forty-eight hours. The nurses told us that according to the "book," patients with a surgery like Ryan's usually had the pressures stabilize by that magical forty-eight hours. When I spoke with the day nurse in charge of Ryan, she kept referring to the "book." Apparently, she did not realize that Ryan had not read the "book" and as such, he was blazing his own trail through recovery. As the events of the day unfolded, we became aware that he was not going to follow the "normal" recovery steps.

As I spoke with one of the nurses, I noticed that she was hedging her answers behind the "book" a lot of the time. I finally confronted her with a question that she did not want to answer; however, I compelled her to tell me the truth. I had spoken with that nurse on several occasions over the days that Ryan had been in PICU and we had a good rapport. I asked her if there was something I should know. "Please tell me if there is something for which I need to prepare my family." After some persuasive discussion on my part, she began to reveal what she had been hearing.

There are two sets of information in a critical care case. There is the information that the doctors give the family and then there is the rest of the information that is shared with the medical staff. I told the nurse that I realized that we did not have all of the details that she did, but I asked her to share with me the information that we needed to have. I shared with her what the doctors had been telling us. She mulled over this information for a moment and then filled in some details based on what she had heard. Part of what I told her was that the original surgeon had told us the mass had been a cancerous tumor. I also explained he had not given us any further information about the type or severity of cancer. I said the doctor had told us were waiting on the pathology report before they gave any more details. They did not want to speculate on the type or possible treatment. We understood that depending on the type of cancer and the severity of it, the course of treatment was vastly different. During my part of the conversation, she nodded her head along with everything I said. She expressed she had been given the same information about the mass being cancerous. She explained her hesitancy to respond to some of my earlier questions because she did not know if the doctor had told the family that it was cancer. I then looked her square in the eye and asked her if she had more information and she looked back at me just as squarely and told me she did have other information. This was both what I wanted to hear and what I feared to hear.

During the conversation that ensued, my world was once again shaken to the core. I was told when they had done the surgery a large portion of the tumor had been left. The doctor had told us a portion of the tumor remained, but he did not elaborate as to how much tumor remained. The nurse explained that the underlying reason that the MRI had been performed on Monday was they wanted to know how much tumor was left behind. Behind "closed doors," the doctors had been discussing the problem of the cranial pressures. According to the nurse, the speculation was that a significant portion of the tumor remained. The concern was the tumor, the fluid accumulation, and the swelling were all combining to leave Ryan in the same condition that he had been in when he arrived at the hospital. Due to the continued problem with stabilizing the cranial pressure, there was talk that a second surgery was inevitable. The surgeon needed to remove the rest of the tumor. The thinking was it was only going to be possible to regulate the pressures if the rest of the tumor was removed. This was not something I wanted to hear, but I had asked for the information. I asked about what the MRI had shown. I was told the MRI had not been read yet. The results of the MRI would play heavily into the decision about doing the second surgery.

I went back to the waiting room and they could tell by the look on my face something was not good. I sat down with them and explained what I had been told. I was uncertain how to process the information I had learned. I wanted to go screaming down the halls that Ryan needed all of the prayers we could gather, but on the other hand we were not sure a second surgery was going to happen so we did not want to get people stirred up if it was not necessary. The stark reality was if Ryan underwent the second surgery, it might help relieve the pressure, but the possibility was very real he would not survive a second surgery. Tuesday morning began at the motel with guarded optimism, but within a very short time after getting to the hospital, that optimism was completely gone. According to the "book," that day was supposed to be the day Ryan started showing improvement and suddenly there was a very real possibility that more surgery was going to happen, quickly.

The doctors had the nurses attempt to raise Ryan's body temperature back to normal on Tuesday morning. The doctors wanted to know how Ryan was going to respond to the warmer temperature. This was the first time in days they were taking positive strides to bring Ryan back to a "normal" state. We knew that it was possible his pressures would go awry and the whole process of adjusting all of the medicines would start again. The cooling blanket was adjusted and we waited. Ryan's pressures did fluctuate; however, they could administer the medications and bring the pressures back in line. We began to think that perhaps the worst was behind us. If they could raise Ryan's body temperature without a major incident, then there really were no boundaries to what could be accomplished in his recovery.

At some point near midday, Ashtyn and Andrea went in to check on Ryan. Ashtyn started rubbing lotion on Ryan's arms and talking to him. Suddenly, Ryan's pulse rate, ICP and CPP all started going in different directions at the same time. They were rushed from the room and the nurses began immediate corrective actions to bring him back in line. This was the second time that this sort of reaction had happened and Andrea had been in the room both times it happened. When the nurses got Ryan to a point that they felt was satisfactory, a nurse talked with Andrea.

None of the medical staff could say with certainty what had caused Ryan's reaction, but they did speculate. They began to theorize that since Ryan and Ashtyn were so close to each other, Ryan was subconsciously trying to call out to his Sissy for help. The nurses seemed to think that even though Ryan was unconscious and in a medically induced coma, he could hear Ashtyn's voice and was trying to get her to help him. His mind knew she was there even though his body could not acknowledge that fact. The advice we were given was exceptionally disturbing. Andrea was told that Ashtyn should be kept away from Ryan. When the nurse realized that Andrea had been present on both occasions, she revised her initial statement about Ashtyn to include everyone. At that point, we were all banned from stimulating Ryan. We could not touch him, we could not speak to him, and we could not let him know we were in the room with him. The nurse told us she knew it was tough, but it was for Ryan's benefit that we had to abide by that rule or we could not go into his room. Andrea returned to the waiting room and she melted into a chair. She began to explain the new rules for going into Ryan's room to the rest of us. This was yet another heart-wrenching episode in this entire saga. The ones who were closest to Ryan were now told we could not talk to him or touch him; all we could do was stand and look at him.

Throughout the afternoon, we kept trying to prepare ourselves for the possibility, which appeared to be becoming more of a probability than a possibility, that a second evacuation procedure would be performed in the very near future. Ryan's pressures kept spiking, sometimes to very high levels. I would watch the numbers and just stand in numbed shock. I could not really get my mind around the fact that though Ryan should have been getting better this day, we were being told of the possibility of another surgery. As we continued to monitor Ryan's progress throughout the day, his pressures just kept bouncing all over the place. The staff was performing at such a high level that we could not ask for better care. It was not their fault that Ryan had failed to read the "book" on how he was supposed to be recovering.

As we waited throughout the day on Tuesday, we kept in the back of our minds Ryan's teacher, Mrs. Kennemer, was going to visit from Pea Ridge on Wednesday. Mrs. Kennemer was bringing Audra, a neighbor of Chris and Andrea's, with her. Chris and Andrea had decided that due to the problems that had been encountered that afternoon with Ryan spiking his pressures when Ashtyn tried to communicate with him, they needed to remove Ashtyn from the hospital setting rather than continually telling her she couldn't go to his room. After all, she was only nine and she loved her little brother. It seemed cruel to tell her that she could not go into his room and see him. Andrea had called and talked to Audra and asked if Ashtyn could stay at Audra's house for a while. Audra readily agreed and so the plans were put into motion. Audra and Mrs. Kennemer would drive to Little Rock to check on Ryan and the rest of the family and then return to Pea Ridge with Ashtyn, who would stay at Audra's house until either Chris or Andrea, or both, returned home. It didn't look like that would be in the near future, certainly not both of them returning home. If they both returned home at that point, it would have only been for one reason, and none of us wanted to plan on them both returning home in the near future.

Pea Ridge is a small town in northwestern Arkansas, and it had not taken long for Ryan's plight to be disseminated throughout the area. One thing that can still be counted on in a day and time when people are always complaining about the state of our country: there are good people who will do whatever is within their power to ease the discomfort of those in need. The community of Pea Ridge made Ryan's case a project for the community to reach out in whatever ways they could.

Shortly after working out the arrangements to get Ashtyn back to Pea Ridge, Andrea received word that a room had become available in the Ronald McDonald House (RMH) starting on Wednesday. Getting a room in the RMH was somewhat bittersweet. The number of rooms was limited, so it was actually quite difficult to get into one of the rooms. It was a blessing that they had been accepted. Unfortunately, room assignments were prioritized, in large part, by the severity of the patient in the hospital. If a patient was not seriously ill, the parents were less likely to get a room than the parents of a more seriously ill patient. Sadly, at the time a room came open, Ryan was moved to the front of the line in almost every category of treatment. I believe that at this time, he was the most critical patient in the PICU. More sadly still, that would not remain the case for very long.

The RMH was a block away from the hospital. Security patrols drove around the hospital all hours of the day and night. When someone was staying in the RMH, they could contact the patrol for a ride to the hospital. Security would pick the parent up at the front door of the house and drop them off at the hospital front door. When the parents wanted to leave the hospital, they would reverse the route to take them home. This was an ideal solution for Andrea so she would not need to try getting back and forth by herself. Security frowned on people, especially women, walking around outside of the hospital unattended. Early in the morning or late at night were especially risky times as criminal activity was a common problem in the neighborhoods around the hospital. Getting a room in the RMH helped alleviate this problem before it really ever began. Without having to stay in a motel and navigate by herself, Andrea could come and go from the hospital at her discretion and have a security escort to do so. The cost of the house was minimal as well. Being unsure of how long the stay in the hospital would be and not knowing how the insurance would work throughout this whole ordeal was a concern. The RMH helped avoid placing an extra financial burden on the families of patients. Even at a discounted rate in a motel, it adds up to a sizable sum very rapidly. Being accepted into the RMH was a great blessing as it solved many problems all at once.

We stumbled through the day, wandering in and out of the unit. Ryan still was not moving because they kept him sedated and paralyzed even though they were warming his body. As his temperature rose, his pressures started to go haywire. We could not bring ourselves to publicize the danger he was facing, so we kept the concern off the website. As Ryan continued to bounce between acceptable numbers and dangerous numbers, the talk turned more and more to a certainty they were going to have to do a second surgery. There seemed to be a consensus, among the nurses, that the second surgery was going to happen and probably as early as Thursday.

We found out the final decision on whether or not Ryan would have the second surgery would be made by the hospital's head neurosurgeon. He had been out of town when the first surgery had been performed, so we did not know him. He had returned to the hospital on Tuesday and one of the first things he was supposed to do was to give a consult on Ryan's case. We did not know anything about him, so I asked the day nurse I knew best about him.

"I have worked here nearly fifteen years and I have worked with a lot of doctors. If I had to trust one doctor with my life, he would be the one," she told me.

After the shifts changed, I began to talk with one of the night shift nurses that I had gotten to know a little bit. I mentioned the conversation about the doctor that I had with the day shift nurse, included the day nurse's response to my questions. The night shift nurse gave me a hearty confirmation that she completely agreed with the day shift nurse. We might not have known the doctor, but we did receive some glowing recommendations from the nursing staff. That at least was a bit of a comfort.

As the day began to wind down Ryan's condition had not improved much. He was still bouncing around on his blood pressure and his cranial pressures. The decision was made to start the cooling blanket treatment again. However, when they tried to cool him to the point at which he had previously been held, around 90°F, he fought the temperature drop, instead of helping his pressures, it caused them to go the wrong way. His ICP spiked and his CPP dropped. They began to raise the temperature of the blanket. When Ryan's body temperature reached 95°F, his pressures leveled out. When his temperature had been back to normal, the pressures had been out of line. The nurses decided to keep the machine set so that Ryan's temperature was 95°F. If it got outside of about a one-half degree range, Ryan's pressures started becoming more unmanageable. When they kept it within that range, they could control his pressures. They were a little surprised because the normal process was to keep the patient as cool as possible. Ryan wouldn't tolerate that cold, so they stopped trying to make that work. By evening, for the first time in days, Ryan's temperature, ICP, CPP, blood pressure, and pulse rate were all in a range that was determined to be acceptable. The readings did not stay that way for very long, but they did seem to be easier to stabilize while they had Ryan's temperature at that 95°F target.

Chris, Jenti, and I were raised by parents who were Christians. We grew up going to church as a family each Sunday. We kids were never sent to church; we were taken. It was instilled in us from our earliest memories that there was a God and that He loved us. We learned about Jesus Christ and the sacrifice of Himself on our behalf. As I had watched Chris through the days and hours, I knew that he would have gladly taken Ryan's place if it had restored Ryan's health. That was not possible. All Chris could do was sit and wait with the rest of us. I knew Chris had faith in Jesus Christ as his Savior, but he was rather closed mouth about his personal testimony. I understood. I had been a Christian for years and it had not been something I was comfortable talking about for most of those years. I think this is a common difficulty for many Christians, but especially for men who are Christians. We do not like to share our feelings and emotions. It is hard to declare our reliance on God. It is hard to admit that we are not able to do something. Chris had been in management for years. It was easy for him to tell people what to do and they did it. He was cordial and hard working and expected those around him to have the same qualities.

Sometimes it caused him problems; he expected more from his workers than they were willing to offer. He did not ask anything that he was not willing to give himself. He was in charge and the workers knew that. He had come to realize that he was far from being in charge in this case. Chris never tried to get up in God's face about why this was happening. He did begin, however, to humble himself before God and admit that God was in control. Chris realized there was nothing he could do, except turn the situation over to God.

It became apparent by Tuesday night that Chris had come to realize that Ryan's life was out of our hands. Ryan's care was in the doctors and nurses hands, but God was in control of them. Once we all accepted the chain of command, life became much easier to face. We did not know what Wednesday would hold. We did not know what the doctors' meeting would decide. What we did know was that Ryan had survived another day and God had been gracious enough to provide a place for Andrea to stay.

Tuesday had been another taxing day. We had received the good news that Andrea would get a place to stay, with a real bed to sleep in the next day. However, we had also received the disturbing news that a second surgery was more than likely in the immediate future. A panel of doctors was to meet on Wednesday morning and discuss what the course of treatment would be. We knew by sometime Wednesday, we would have the decision about whether or not a surgery was to be performed. We stayed at the hospital until 9:00 p.m. and right on schedule the cleaning crew came in and started making us feel uneasy about still being in the waiting room. Ashtyn had gone home with Mames on Tuesday evening, so it was just Nonna, Poppa, and me. Our little band of hospital pilgrims was dwindling, but that was okay. Life had to continue; there was nothing that could be gained by everyone continually sitting in the waiting room. Each of us had to return to our own lives at some point in time.

Tuesday's hospital stay for us ended. Nonna, Poppa, and I headed back to the motel, stretched out across the beds, and turned on the TV. This was the first time we had bothered to turn the silly thing on in the days we had been at the motel. It did not work properly and was all sorts of weird colors. It did not matter; we were not interested in keeping up with the show. We just needed something mindless playing for a diversion. Tuesday had been bad and we knew that Wednesday could be worse. Trying to stay positive was getting more and more difficult. Fortunately, I was so exhausted that sleep came more quickly than normal and I was lost to the nightmare we were living, at least for a while.

Wednesday morning dawned much the same way it had for the previous few days. Nonna, Poppa, and I all got ready and headed for the hospital. We got there right at 9:00 a.m., which had become our routine. When Nonna, Poppa, and I got to the hospital, I went to check on Ryan while Nonna and Poppa talked to Chris. I hadn't talked to Chris, so I was in for a big shock when I got to Ryan's room. The doorway into Ryan's room had two doors. There was the big door, which was a standard thirty-six inch door and there was a smaller door, which opened the opposite direction. The design allowed the doorway to convert from a regular door to extra wide door, for moving equipment or beds in and out of the room. When we got to the hospital on Wednesday morning, the large door was closed and a desk had been moved in front it. The large door had been closed to keep the room as quite and stimuli free as possible. Having the large door closed kept a large portion of the ambient background noise of the PICU from entering into the room. The lights were turned almost completely off; only one bank of lights remained lit. The small door was the only way in and out of Ryan's room and there was a note on the door that told everyone that Ryan needed as little stimulation as possible. The note reminded us we needed to be completely quiet and to refrain from touching Ryan.

After days of bad news, I think walking into that scenario was probably the proverbial "straw that broke the camel's back." Ryan's pressures were not holding acceptable, the possibility was very great that Ryan was going to have a second surgery in the very near future, and to top it off we now found out we were not allowed to try to touch or speak to Ryan as this was contributing to the problems. The situation had not changed, but the scene with the minimized door opening and the sign on the door, seemed to indicate we were somehow part of the problem in Ryan's condition. Those words were not spoken, but the sentiment seemed to be very clear: if we would just leave him alone, he would be better off.

Chris came into the room while I was standing over Ryan's bed praying for him again. He told me in a whisper, "The respiratory therapist believes Ryan is developing pneumonia. They are going to increase the breathing treatments from every six hours to every four hours." I looked into his haggard face and I noticed a greater degree of sadness in Chris' eyes than I had seen before. He turned around and squeezed out the narrow doorway. I finished praying for Ryan and I too left the room and headed for the waiting room.

Rather than risk stimulating Ryan, we all spent a major portion of the morning in the waiting room. We were all numb, practically beyond description. Our hopes had been continually dashed upon the shores of reality. Every time we thought Ryan was going to stabilize, something else happened which seemed to make the situation more dire. One of our main sources of encouragement and inspiration was the CaringBridge guestbook. As people would write words of encouragement and let us know they were praying for us, it offered the consolation we were being lifted up in prayer.

There began to be a sense of urgency in getting the prayer map completed. The prayer map was something that was continually hanging on the wall in Ryan's room, unless it was actively being updated. All of the doctors and nurses knew what that map stood for, and they continued to encourage us to reach out in support of prayer and inspiration. As each day passed and Ryan's condition did not improve, the staff was well aware that Ryan might never wake from his chemically induced coma. I never had anyone tell me that Ryan might die, but it was obvious from the comments that were made that none of the staff would have been surprised if he had. That was never a part of any discussion I was a part of, at least not that I could remember; however, it was a constant source of angst within my own heart. I longed to see the little man's eyes opened again, to see him laugh again, even to see him pout. The prayers of all God's children were, I believe, what saw us through this darkest of hours. We were helpless, unable to comfort him or to speed his recovery. Rock bottom would be the location I would say we were pretty much all at by mid-morning Wednesday. Tensions were mounting as we were still awaiting the results of the doctor's meeting.

As it approached noon, Mrs. Kennemer and Audra arrived at the hospital. They had driven to Little Rock from Pea Ridge that morning. They wanted to check on the family and see how they were doing and Mrs. Kennemer was very set on getting to see "her" Ryan. Unbeknownst to me at that time, this was not the first time she had dealt with one of her students having a life-threatening crisis. She truly had a passion for her students, and her dedication and determination to be there for Ryan and family was a boost just when it was most needed. When she and Audra arrived, the tide of anguish seemed to be stemmed for a bit. Here were people from "home." Teacher and neighbor, arriving and bringing with them more offerings of compassion from those around the town of Pea Ridge and from the school where Ryan and Ashtyn both attended. Food items, activities, toys, cash, all things that were very useful were presented. Assurances that people were doing all they could behind the scenes to cover every possible thing that could be handled.

A sense of peace seemed to rest over us for a while as talk turned to home and the future. Andrea and Audra talked about things that needed handled in the Mondy home back in Pea Ridge. Mrs. Kennemer reminisced about her memories of Ryan in her class. She talked of plans for his future and his education. She spoke of his classmates' desire to have him return. She spoke plainly of the faith of the children. They did not understand the gravity of the situation, but they did have the love and faith of children. They had sent Ryan pictures and cards, and they let everyone know they had no doubts Ryan would join them once again, they were just anxious to have it happen as soon as possible.

Suddenly, as we spoke with Mrs. Kennemer and Audra, the floodgates of Heaven were opened and God's mercy and grace began to rain down upon us in Biblical flood-like proportions. The doctor's board concluded its meeting. Chris and Andrea were called in to speak with the doctors and when they returned to the waiting room, we received the best news we had heard since Ryan's diagnosis. The doctors decided a second surgery was not to be performed. As the doctors had studied the MRI, they had determined the majority of the tumor had been removed. The neurosurgeon explained that a "rind" of the tumor was all that remained. The "rind" was the portion of the tumor that was directly affixed to the brain. The surgeon had left the portion closest to the brain, mostly because of the instrumentation problem they had encountered. The decision made by the board was if another surgery was performed, it could cause more problems with Ryan's motor skills and cause further damage to his ability to use his left side.

Instead of trying to do surgery, the doctors had decided they would wait for the pathology report to return from the three labs to which biopsy samples had been sent. When the reports were all compiled and an oncology result was known, the tumor would be treated as deemed best. A second surgery was not in the immediate future and the ground that Ryan was trying to gain in his recovery would not be hindered by any further surgery at this time.

According to the MRI, the void left from the tumor removal was indeed full of fluid. The doctors told Chris and Andrea that as Ryan's body realized this fluid was not supposed to be there, it would start absorbing the fluid into his system. The results of the doctor's meeting left us with the understanding that if Ryan could survive until the pressure could be regulated, he would be on a solid foundation to proceed with the rest of his recovery. The problem was while he was fighting the pressure issues, he was developing pneumonia.

Chris and Andrea were so relieved and overwhelmed at the report from the doctors that they could not respond with a journal update. I sat down, and through tears of joy, I began to write. I wrote all of the things that had been relayed to us. Ryan did not have to have a second surgery; he was making progress even though it seemed as if he was getting continually worse.

For the first time in almost six days, since the original diagnosis on November 3, we had hope. We had been given the assurance that Ryan's determination was a key in his recovery. If he were willing to fight, he would get better quicker. At that time, we knew he had a stubborn streak, but nobody could have envisioned his amazing attitude and ability.

We still could not talk to him or touch him, but we knew he was many days closer to waking up than he would be if he had undergone the second surgery. Chris and Andrea talked with the doctors about the restrictions of no touching or talking to Ryan. The doctors explained it something like this: Ryan's body was paralyzed by chemicals, and he could not move. He was on high levels of painkillers and sedatives to keep him from experiencing the pain. However, his brain was still functioning, at least on a subconscious level. It was much like being in a very sound sleep, apparently. He was not awake and actively responding to stimuli, but at the same time, his brain was not "turned off." His body was capable of hearing sounds and his subconscious was processing those sounds. When his body was touched, his nerves processed the stimuli and told his brain something was happening.

As we began to understand what was going on more and more, it caused a sense of overwhelming dismay in Nonna. All she could envision was Ryan trapped inside of his body. She could not bear the thought of Ryan being able to experience any of this. We kept assuring her that even though he was dealing with it in his subconscious; he could not feel the pain. It was a very difficult thing to process for all of us, but it hit her very hard. We flew through the rest of Wednesday, but that night brought one of the funniest events that would happen through this entire ordeal.

Chris and Andrea had lived in Utah for a few years. In mid-2005, Chris changed positions within the company he worked for and was able to move back to Arkansas. In October of 2005, I flew to Utah so I could help them move back. Andrea flew, with the kids, to St. Louis, Missouri, where Nonna and Poppa met them and they traveled from St. Louis to Pea Ridge. On the other end, Chris and I began the journey across country with each of us driving one of their vehicles. I had agreed that I would be glad to help if he would provide me with food and a place to sleep each night. For him that sounded like a good trade-off because it kept him from having to make the trip two times by himself.

We would drive most of the day, stopping for something quick and light for lunch and keep driving. By the time evenings rolled around, were extremely hungry. On the second full day of travel, we made it to St. Joseph, Missouri. We were going to spend the night with our cousin in Kansas City, Missouri, that night, so we decided to stop for supper in St. Joseph before heading on into Kansas City for the night.

We stopped at a Red Lobster and went in to eat. Our faces began to glow as the waiter told us the special was their "endless shrimp" sale. We could eat all of the shrimp we wanted for one price. We looked at each other and smiled. It was time to get our, Chris', money's worth. After several refills, we joked around with the server about how much we were eating. He told us he had served two teenage girls who had ordered and eaten 180 scampi each. We told him we wished he had told us that in advance, we would have tried to break that mark. As it was, we had several refills, but we could not verify how many shrimp we had eaten. When the check came, the refills were listed and the ticket was about 18 inches long.

After we concluded our delicious meal at Red Lobster, we went to our Cousin Amy's house where we regaled them with what appeared to be quite the "fish story." Amy's husband, also named Chris, found it extremely funny and when my brother Chris pulled the receipt out that made the story that much more funny.

Now here we were again, my brother and I on a journey together… and we were hungry! Chris decided that he wanted to eat at Red Lobster; and as you might have guessed, "endless shrimp" was once again the special. We were tired, stressed, and most of all, hungry. As we sat down memories of what we had done the previous year came to the surface and we began to laugh and remember. Chris called our cousin's house and talked to Cousin Chris. He told our cousin we were getting ready to eat all of the shrimp we could. All three of us began to laugh, and for a time the problems seemed to be staved off. Good food and laughter seem to have a soothing effect on our family.

The server came to our table to take our order. "What can I get you tonight?"

"Ma'am," I began, "we have been sitting in the hospital waiting room all day, and we are hungry. We are going to have the endless shrimp, and we are going to eat a scary amount of it."

She chuckled, "I have seen big eaters before, and I think we can handle it."

Before the meal was done, that chuckle turned to quiet amazement, then to something that resembled fear. I don't know if she was afraid we would be sick, or perhaps, she was afraid of being bit if she got too close.

We had a goal in mind when we began the meal. We wanted to beat the mark that had been set by the two teenage girls we had heard about the previous year. I began a tally sheet to try to keep track of how many we ate. The entrée portions came and we told the server to go ahead and get refills. By the time she brought the first refill, we had eaten the original portions of shrimp. We asked if she could get two refills each, to cut down on the wait time. She said she had been told she could not place a refill order until after she had delivered the previous refill. We told her to keep them coming as quickly as possible. See, we had been told you could only eat for twenty minutes before your body realizes it is getting full. We did not want to realize we were too full before we made our goal.

I must say we had an excellent server. The scampi came on a regular basis. The sauce on the scampi would still be bubbling when they arrived. The dishes they cook the scampi in are cast iron and the refills would be so hot that the shrimp sizzled. The shrimp were so hot that our fingers got sore from holding the tails to eat the shrimp. I kept switching hands because my fingers got so sore I could not hold onto the shrimp. That twenty-minute thing, I am not sure how accurate it is. We ate scampi for a solid 45 minutes, just as hot as we could stand it. By the time the server could get a refill to the table, the previous one was empty.

Then it happened. Chris leaned back and said, "Uncle." He could not hold anymore. I just smiled and told the server to keep it coming. I have always been a big eater, and I was having fun. Finally, I called it quits also. I had eaten two cheddar biscuits, my salad, and my order of garlic-mashed potatoes in addition to my scampi. Chris had bailed out; he had picked at his salad and only eaten part of his potatoes and had stopped before me. We were satisfied and ready for the check. I had kept track of how many refills we had each had and we had each passed

our previous mark. We got the ticket and I found out I had forgotten to
write down one refill each. So there it was. We had eaten more scampi
than before and feeling quite proud of our accomplishment. Then we
began to laugh because we calculated how much each of the shrimp had
actually cost. We figured out that shrimp at Red Lobster was very
inexpensive if we got the "endless shrimp" and really did eat a near
endless amount. Before the tip, it worked out to about $0.075 per
shrimp, and that was having Red Lobster prepare them for us. Between
the two of us, we had cleaned out 330 shrimp scampi that evening. It
turned out to be less than the girls ate, but we had done our best.

The laughter didn't just fade away into the night. For the first time
since the ordeal began, there was good news. Ryan was not to have the
surgery, Andrea and Nonna were going to spend the night in the RMH,
and the "Nation of Prayer Map" had showed prayer support in thirty-
nine states. Hope had begun to shine brighter and our confidence level
had risen as the day progressed. Wednesday night we were not just
gorging ourselves, we were celebrating in a way. Ryan was on the
mend and the doctors had confirmed that information.

Yes, it seemed that as dark as the forecast had been the night
before, rays of light were illuminating the future. Little did we know
what Thursday morning held in store for all of us. Just when we
believed that Ryan was stabilizing and starting to gain ground, just as
we started to see light at the end of the tunnel, just as we were starting to
become more at ease, then we were blindsided one more time.

Sometimes the littlest of things can cause the greatest uproar. As
Wednesday ended, we were unaware of the turmoil that waited to
pounce on us Thursday. We each slept that evening with a calming
knowledge Ryan did not need that second surgery, at least not now.
Chris and I had eaten ourselves into a scampi stupor. We had laughed
and enjoyed our time together. I lay down Wednesday night with a
knowledge that my wife, Laura, was flying to Little Rock on Thursday
evening. Wednesday ended more peacefully than the nights before. As
I fell asleep, I remember thinking about how I was actually looking
forward to what was to come on Thursday. Little did I know that it
would be one of the most trying days yet.

Thursday dawned with just Poppa and me at the motel. I got up
and headed to the hospital, Poppa stayed around the room getting his
stuff ready to go home on that day. He was going to go home and Laura
was flying in that evening. I was very anxious to see my wife. I had
been in the midst of this maelstrom from the beginning and I very much
wanted to have her by my side.

When I got to the PICU waiting room, Nonna and Andrea were there. Andrea appeared extremely upset. Chris walked into the waiting room at the same time I did. He had been in Ryan's room and he didn't seem upset. I was perplexed as to why Andrea was so distraught. Chris sat down in a chair and Andrea sat down on his lap, dropped her head onto his shoulder, and began weeping uncontrollably. I looked to Chris and he was just as puzzled as I was.

Andrea had been so strong through this entire ordeal. She had talked with me at great lengths a couple of nights earlier, as she was putting stuff in the van. We had stood in the parking lot and talked for close to an hour. She was very much upset about Ryan's condition and she had many common questions about whether or not she should have done something more and caught Ryan's tumor sooner. We talked and talked and I did my best to assure her at that point, and I reiterate it here. I think Andrea is a great mom who cares for children and her husband very much. I did not believe there was one thing that could have been done differently. I told her when Ryan was sick, she had taken him to the doctor. If the doctor had not been able to detect this tumor earlier, then she certainly could not expect to have known it any sooner either. As we talked, she became more emotional than she had in the days leading up to this talk, but on Thursday morning, she became a total basket case.

"Honey, what's wrong," Chris tried to comfort her.

"Ashtyn has head lice!" she wailed.

Chris looked like a deer caught in someone's headlights. He did not know which way to turn and he did not know what to say. He put his arms around her and drew her closer into him. She sobbed on his shoulder for a few minutes, and then she began to tell us the story.

"Audra called me just before we left the house to come to the hospital. Ashtyn went to school this morning and while she was there, she began scratching her head. The school nurse checked her and she had head lice. The school called Audra and she had to go to school and pick Ashtyn up and take her home. She had live lice crawling on her scalp."

Simultaneously we all reached up and began scratching our heads. We must have looked like a bunch of apes, checking each other for lice. The problem was that none of us knew what we were looking for. Of course, we began talking in subdued tones after that initial outburst by Andrea. We did not want the other people in the waiting room to find out what we were so secretly discussing.

The concerns about head lice jumped to the forefront of our day. We discussed the possibility of where Ashtyn could have gotten the lice. She had been playing in the play area of the hospital over the past few days. She had been to Mames' house and spent the night there on Tuesday, just before going home with Audra. She had been to the RMH, but she had not slept there, though she had been given a stuffed animal. While she played with the bear, she hugged it and every place it touched her face, her skin turned red. We wondered if it could have been infested.

Ashtyn having head lice was bad, but worse yet, if Andrea or Nonna had lice, they would have to give up their room at the RMH. None of us had ever dealt with head lice before, so we did the only thing that we could do. Andrea discussed the situation with one of the social workers at the hospital and the social worker had a nurse check out Andrea and Nonna. Chris and I had very short hair, so we were not concerned. Andrea and Nonna were lice free, so whatever had happened, all of the adults were free of lice.

As we continued to discuss the situation, Andrea grew afraid that Ashtyn might have contaminated Ryan the last time she was in his room. In the midst of the discussion, Audra called back and told Andrea that they had gotten the lice shampoo and washed Ashtyn's hair, but that there were still lice crawling in her hair.

Andrea got very upset again. One child is laying in PICU on death's doorstep and the other one was miles away dealing with another condition. Andrea felt like a failure as a mother because there was nothing she could do for either one of her children. She was trapped in a land, which bred futility. My heart ached for Andrea. Just when things were beginning to seem like Ryan was making a positive turn, this struck.

Audra called the school nurse to find out what she should do since the shampoo hadn't worked. The nurse recommended that Audra soak Ashtyn's hair in olive oil, wrap plastic wrap around her hair, and leave it for a minimum of three hours. The nurse said that this would smother any live lice that might be remaining. As Audra had a little girl with whom Ashtyn had been playing the night before, Audra applied the treatment to both girls at the same time. As the girls sat with their hair soaked in olive oil and wrapped in plastic wrap, Audra washed all of the bedclothes and the girls' clothing. To speed up the washing process, she used her washing machine and the one in Chris and Andrea's home. She ran back and forth from house to house doing all of the laundry.

Nonna called her sister, Lisa, and talked to her about the situation. When she called Lisa, Lisa began to laugh aloud. Nonna did not think it was very funny, and Andrea was incensed. Lisa reminded them that head lice are a common ailment among children.

Lisa quipped, "You may not be able to do anything about Ryan's condition, but life is going to return to normal. The head lice are just a sign from God that normalcy reigns and extraordinary circumstances will return to normal some day."

While Nonna and Andrea went on a nit-hunt, I went around to Ryan's room. My head was crawling at this point, but as I said before, I had very short hair and it was obvious that I did not have anything about which to be concerned. I spoke with the day nurse, and then I went back to the waiting room and told everyone what had happened. Poppa had gotten to the hospital, but he was getting ready to head for home. I wanted to make sure he was as up to date as possible before he left.

"Ryan's ICP has been holding stable in the single digits. His CPP is strong and holding stable also." I continued, "As I was talking to the nurse, she was trying to give him a sponge bath. While she was working on him, his blood pressure shot up to 160/100. When the monitor sounded, she stepped back and left Ryan alone for a few minutes. His blood pressure dropped back to 135/85. While his blood pressure was up, I watched his ICP reading and it remained stable."

It may seem like a small incident, but what it indicated was that Ryan's body had finally begun to handle stress, as it should. He was definitely getting better. His ICP staying down was the absolute best news for which we could hope. His heart racing did present a concern though. I informed his doctor of a condition that I had and gave him a bit of family history relevant to that condition so they could check Ryan for the condition. When I shared the information with the doctor, he saw my concern and assured me that they would definitely check into it. After the tests had been done, it was determined that Ryan's heart was perfectly normal. The racing of his heart was just a response to stimuli.

The turmoil over the head lice had died down somewhat since it was first brought to light. Andrea and Nonna were clear, that meant that the McDonald House was OK because Ashtyn had not stayed there. I, on the other hand, was concerned because I had taken a feather mattress with me in case someone needed a place to sleep. Ashtyn had used it for a few nights before she left, and then when she left, I spread it across my bed to add a little more cushion. I decided that I needed to make sure there was no lice in the motel before Laura got to Little Rock.

It is somewhat strange that as much as we had worried and fretted over Ryan's condition for days and days, it took something as small as lice to get our attentions off him for a while as we scurried to try to get everything righted. I guess when Lisa had laughed about the lice it had changed our perspective a bit. When there is absolutely nothing one can do except trust God, then there is no reason to try to do anything more. However, when there is something that needs to be done, something, which we can do, we really should be faithful in doing those things. I think the greatest lesson I learned that day was that my responsibility really lies in being able to determine the difference in those two types of things. Do what I can do, but trust God when it is beyond me. Sounds simple, but you would be amazed at how many people still have a God complex and think that they have to be actively involved to help God get the job done. Sometimes He uses us, but we really need to be certain that He wants our help. If He wants us to just wait for Him to work, we are greatly benefited if we just wait on Him. I really began to focus on this lesson, but it would take a few more weeks before I really got my eyes opened.

Shortly after I knew that I had the room de-contaminated, Laura's plane arrived. I headed to the airport to pick her up. Her plane was right on schedule. She arrived shortly before visiting hours were supposed to end, so we decided to wait on dinner and we went straight to the hospital so she could see Ryan. I had text messaged a picture of Ryan to her earlier in the week, so she knew what she was walking into when she got there. Even advance knowledge did not make entering the room easier. When Laura got to Little Rock, the nurse was still keeping the room darkened and the noise to a minimum. The big door was still closed and the sign remained on the doorway. I went into the room with her and we discussed Ryan in hushed tones as I tried to answer her questions about the monitors and the readings.

She did not get to stay for very long because visiting hours were ending. We got Andrea and Nonna together, took them to the McDonald House, and dropped them off. Finally, about 10:00 p.m. Laura and I were able to eat. As we talked about Ryan and about how things had been going at our house the previous week, I began to realize just how truly bone-tired I was. We finished eating and went back to the motel to get some rest.

I went to sleep that evening wondering just how long we could continue at that pace. Would we burn out, or would we be able to withstand the time factor and see this through? I was tired, but Chris was not getting the amount of rest I was getting. I could not imagine how he continued to put one foot in front of the other as the days passed.

Friday morning came, and with it another trip to the hospital. I found that Thursday night had been a replay of the previous days and nights, still struggling to keep the pressures in a normal range. They had struggled through the night to maintain his body temperature at that mystical 95°F. The problem was that it was very difficult to keep that tight of a range. Apparently, the developing pneumonia was causing a fever. As his body was forcing his temperature to go up, they had to use the cooling blanket largely to bring his temperature down. During the blanket's cycle, it caused Ryan to cool down below his desired temperature and it caused pressure fluctuations. The ICP spikes were not as dramatic, but they were still hitting a level that concerned the doctor.

I knew this would be my last full day in Little Rock, as I had to head home on Saturday. I think when Laura got to the hospital on Thursday night the dynamic of the situation changed. With her there, everyone realized I would soon be leaving. We had talked about her coming for days; however, the discussions were all in the future tense. When she arrived in Little Rock, it signaled a passing of time. What had once been future suddenly became present.

I really began to wonder if I could leave the hospital the next day. However, Laura had to get home so she could go to work on Monday. I had already missed one week of services. I felt I really needed to be back to preach on Sunday. We had hemmed ourselves into a timetable, which meant we would have to leave on Saturday.

Laura and I went around to the PICU so we could check on Ryan. There had been problems with Ryan's temperature, blood pressure, heart rate, ICP and CPP all the way through. The pneumonia had been a late addition to the crisis. When I spoke with the nurse, I found out the concern over Ryan's lungs had jumped to the front of the line as far as danger went. I began to be very concerned about the situation, but I had a valid reason for concern.

As a pastor, I spend a lot of time around hospitals. I had known a man who had undergone open-heart surgery the previous year. The day after his surgery, I had visited him. He was awake and they had even had him on his feet by the time I spoke with him. Within twenty-four hours after I visited him, he began to have complications. They sedated him, and ended up placing him in a chemically induced coma, the same type Ryan had been in for days. His body rapidly moved from just a heart problem to a heart problem with a side complication of pneumonia. His heart began to regulate; however, they kept him in the chemically induced coma for nearly a week and tried to cure the pneumonia before awakening him. His heart progressed acceptably, but his lungs got weaker with each passing day. Seven days after surgery, he passed away from pneumonia.

As I remembered the situation with the man I had known and called on, I could not help but draw parallels with Ryan. He was at about the same time post operation as this man had been, and now Ryan was developing more and more problems with his lungs. The thing that Ryan did have on his side was that he was very young and had healthy lungs. The man I had known before had been retired for many years and had a history of health problems. I just hoped and prayed the age difference and the overall health differences would be enough to stave off further complications.

Before we arrived at the hospital that morning, the respiratory therapist had conferred with the neurology doctors. Jointly, they determined the best treatment for Ryan's lungs was a more invasive treatment than had been performed previously. Instead of using the external massager, they began to use a technique where bursts of air were pulsed, through one of the ventilator tubes, directly into Ryan's lungs. A separate tube was then utilized to suction the mucus out. The hope was his pressures and rates would be stable enough to work on his lungs. In addition to the new therapy, Ryan's antibiotic regimen had changed also. While we were informed about the change in treatment, we were told we needed to vacate the room so they could work with him for a bit. Having to leave the room that time was not all bad though. We were told we would be able to talk to him and touch him again when they were finished.

As the new breathing treatment was being tried in Ryan's room, we waited in the waiting room. While we waited, a new family came into the waiting room. After a week in the PICU room, we were pretty well acquainted with all of the families that were there. Some were there for just a short while; some had been there all week long with us. Some families received good news, while others got bad news. The new family that came in did not look like there was any good news to be had. Due to privacy laws, we could not get any information from the nurses about what was happening to that family.

Shortly after the new family arrived in the waiting room, we were allowed to return to Ryan's room. As Laura and I went back to see Ryan, Chris spoke with the family to let them know where everything was in the waiting area. He found out this was the extended family of a child being airlifted to ACH. As we entered Ryan's room, we noticed that the large room next to Ryan's was being prepared for the new arrival. The smaller rooms in PICU did not have room for many machines, so we assumed the new patient was in serious condition since he was going into the big room. Some of Ryan's secondary caregivers were being pulled away from his case to start working on preparation for the new arrival. I never heard many details about the child's case, but I do know the child did not survive. He came into the PICU on Friday and was there throughout the afternoon and evening, but he did not survive until I left the next day. I never got a chance to get to know his family. From what I gathered, the child had a brain disorder and had been in and out of the hospital all of his life. On that day, he had collapsed and by the time they got him to the hospital, all brain function had ceased.

Death was a reality that we had avoided talking about as much as possible. We did not want to imagine the worst for Ryan; however, the passing of the little boy in the room next to Ryan's reinforced the reality that children do not always survive health crises. Knowing that Ryan was suffering from multiple life-threatening conditions at one time made us extremely anxious as we watched his little chest heave with every ventilator forced breath.

During the revised respiratory therapy, Ryan's pressures had fluctuated somewhat; however, he had settled back to acceptable readings rather quickly. For the first time in days, the nurse told us we could talk to him, so Laura talked to him a little bit. We had been silent while in his room since she had gotten to Little Rock. She talked with him about being glad to see him. She told him about the people she worked with who were praying for him. She also told him that the people in our church were praying for him and she further elaborated that there were people all around Centralia praying for him. She told him about how they were reading the website to keep up with how he was doing. She had brought him a stuffed dog, and she told him about it as well.

After we checked in on him and spent some time with him, we went back to the waiting room. We talked about Laura and me leaving the next day. We caught up with what had been going on with my kids while I had been gone and we talked about the things coming up in the next week. I could feel myself pulling away from the situation in Little Rock as I began to re-orient myself for the coming week. As we talked, I realized my being in Little Rock had been important to Chris and Andrea, but my attentions were being turned from there to home and the matters for which I was responsible. The longer we talked, the more everyone realized that I was going to leave the next day unless there was some completely unforeseen disaster. Ryan finally appeared to be getting more stable and even though he was still not out of the woods, he was withstanding the more aggressive breathing treatment and our talking with him.

Andrea went in to spend some time with Ryan and when she came back, she told us she had spoken to him and had rubbed his stomach. When she had touched him, his blood pressure and heart rate had both spiked. The readings did not self-regulate, as they needed to, so an additional amount of sedative was given. The nurse told Andrea to pass the word that we could talk to Ryan, but it would be best if we did not touch him yet. The best news to come out of that encounter was that even though his BP and pulse elevated, the ICP did not go up. With the extra sedative, his BP and pulse returned to acceptable.

It seemed as if he had finally turned a corner and was getting better. Our stimulation still had to be held in check, but we could at least speak to him and he was OK with that. They had gotten him regulated on his temperature and his cranial pressures, blood pressure, and heart rate were all holding steady. When he would start to get outside the groove, the nurses would adjust his sedative and he came right back in line. A week into this nightmare and we began to feel as if we could see light at the end of the tunnel. We had been here before though, so no one became overly optimistic. We had learned that patience was the best thing. We knew that at any moment he could turn the other direction; he had done it several times throughout the week. For now, he was settled down, and for that we were thankful.

About 7:00 p.m., we decided it was time for Laura and me to leave for the night. Chris assured me that if anything came up he would call us. I walked out of the hospital. It was only a matter of hours from being one complete week since I had walked into the hospital. Never have I spent a more stressful week. Throughout the week, Ryan had tottered his way down a winding path between life and death. It was dark by the time we left the hospital; it had been dark the week before when I got there. I thought about that for a moment and decided that, metaphorically at least, it had been dark the entire time I had been in Little Rock. I was very glad Laura was with me. I was actually very relieved to be leaving the hospital two full hours before visiting hours ended and knowing that Ryan was more stable at this time than he had been the entire week before.

Laura and I hadn't eaten since lunch, so we decided to get dinner. For the first and probably only time in our lives, we ate ice cream sundaes for dinner. We did not eat even one bite of healthy food for dinner, just some delicious ice cream. We figured that one time wouldn't hurt us and besides, we had learned the hard way that life is too unpredictable not to do the things you truly enjoy occasionally.

We had spent Friday on the most level terrain of the entire week. Ryan had a few difficulties, but overall he had been relatively stable. He had been easier to regulate than any day previous and that gave us the illusion that he was finally on the road to recovery. We had made it through the first week, with all of its difficulties, and we were bracing ourselves for the week to come. Ironically, the day he had been the most stable so far would be the last "stable" day for some time to come.

He's Awake

Saturday morning dawned with a palpable difference. I was going home, regardless of Ryan's condition. I was not sure I was prepared to leave, but I had to go. Since the trip home was about seven hours long and I needed to get home at a decent time, we were going to need to leave by noon.

We got dressed, packed the suitcases, and loaded the van, then went to the hospital for a short visit before we left for home. When we arrived at the hospital, we heard from Chris about how impressed Nurse Valerie had been with Ryan's recovery.

Nurse Valerie had been on duty the Friday night when Ryan had first been admitted. She babied Ryan that night and gave him all the attention he wanted. When he wanted something, she was immediately at his side. He had really taken a liking to her. She had been off all week, as she only worked the weekend shift. In her opinion, Ryan was much better than he had been the previous Saturday night, which had been the last time she had seen him. That thought sent a shiver up my spine. He was still in a chemically induced coma and the pressures inside his head were not stable, but she thought he was much better. That said a lot for how bad he really had been when they admitted him to the hospital. I had seen him the same night she had first seen him. Apparently, she had some information that we did not know that night. As Chris spoke with her through the night hours, she had expressed a little bit of surprise that Ryan had survived the week. When she saw him the second Friday night, she was thrilled to be able to care for him once again.

Laura and I went back to check on Ryan's progress frequently during our final hours in Little Rock that Saturday morning. The latest antibiotics and more aggressive breathing treatments had the pneumonia on the run. Ryan stopped running a fever, so they attempted to turn the chilling blanket off once again. With the chilling blanket off, Ryan's temperature was self-regulating; he warmed to normal body temperature, but did not spike a fever. His pressures were finally holding steady with his body being at its normal temperature. These were exceedingly good signs, so we thought. He was warmer than he had been in days and his pressures were stable. We just kept telling ourselves it was going to take baby steps to get him back. The first step was being warm with stable pressures, and then we would take the next step.

Perhaps, we thought, in a few days they can start to reduce his sedative level and bring him out of the coma. There had been some talk by the doctors that by the middle of the next week they were speculating they would try to awaken Ryan. Everything hinged on how Ryan responded. The doctors did have a rough design for his treatment in mind, but they made hourly adjustments in the plan according to how Ryan responded to each move they made. It was like one huge chess game. For every move the doctors made, Ryan made a countermove.

Laura and I were going home, but Jenti was coming back to Little Rock. She got to the hospital a little while before we headed home. About noon, Laura and I made one last trek to Ryan's room. His temperature was okay and his pressures were still holding where they should. The breathing treatments they had begun the day before were ongoing and it did not seem to be causing problems. We said our goodbyes to Ryan and then we told everyone else goodbye. We gave hugs and kisses around, walked out to the parking lot, and left the hospital. Our lives were going forward; we were hoping that Ryan would go forward with us. We hated to leave, but we had to get started or we would be very late getting home.

We drove for about two hours and had almost made it to West Memphis, Arkansas, before my cell phone rang. I saw on the caller ID that it was Jenti. I answered the phone while I was driving and I wish now I had pulled over to take the call when I heard the words that came out of her mouth.

"He's awake," Jenti gleefully shrieked into my ear.

"Did you just say, 'He's awake'?" I sputtered.

"Yes, I said he is awake," Jenti shot back.

"By 'he', you do mean Ryan don't you?" I clarified.

"Yes, goofy. Ryan is awake. He woke up just a few minutes ago," she bantered. "I have to go. We have a lot of people to call and tell." Then she was gone.

I know I must have looked like someone who had just received the greatest shock of his or her life. I know I looked that way, because I had just received the biggest shock of my life. When Jenti uttered those words, I was more surprised than I had been when I got that original call from Nonna. I had just been there. He was paralyzed; he was sedated; he was on a ventilator. He was on death's doorstep when I left two hours before and now Jenti was calling to tell me "He's awake." I knew it was not a joke. We kid a lot in my family and sometimes we say things that are unkind or perhaps a bit rude. No one was joking about the severity of Ryan's condition and when I heard those words, I knew that as hard as they were to believe, they had to be true.

Mouth agape and utterly speechless, I turned to look at Laura. It was obvious that she had ascertained from my end of the conversation that Ryan had awakened.

"He woke up," I told her.

"I gathered that from your conversation," she beamed. "Do you want to go back and see him?"

"I would love to, but that adds an extra four hours to the trip just to get back to where we are. It would be tomorrow morning before we got home if we did that. As much as I would love to go back, we had better go on home," I reasoned aloud.

I had a sermon to present on Sunday morning, so I needed to get home and get some rest. Instead of turning back toward Little Rock, we continued our journey toward home, but our hearts were soaring far faster than the van was traveling for the rest of that trip.

I had no idea of what had transpired after we left until we reached our home in Illinois. I tried a few times to call someone in Little Rock, but everyone was on the phone spreading the news. I told them I would call when I reached home and they could fill me in on the details. Actually, I got home and checked on the CaringBridge site to see if Chris had updated and then I called him to get the rest of the details. Between the two sources, I received the whole story.

When Ryan's pressures stabilized with his body temperature being normal, the doctors had decided it was time to remove the paralytic, as its primary function was to stop Ryan's body from shivering from the cold. When the cooling blanket was disconnected, the paralytic was not needed. The doctors did not want to keep Ryan on any more medication than was necessary. Everyone had gone to the waiting room to avoid disturbing Ryan with their talking and within a few minutes after they had returned to the waiting area, one of the people working the reception desk rushed in to get a family member. The receptionist did not give them any specifics, only that the nurse had requested a family member right away. Chris and Andrea rushed toward his room and when they walked in, they found him awake. When the paralytic was discontinued, Ryan had fought his way through the sedative and had unexpectedly awakened.

Chris and Andrea talked with Ryan, who was upset because he could not see. There was a thick salve coating his eyes to protect his corneas from exposure to the air. His eyelids would not completely close due to the facial swelling that remained. With his body paralyzed, his eyelids could not blink to keep his eyeballs moist. The salve was liberally applied and it completely sealed the eyeball inside, away from the air.

Trying to divert Ryan's attention away from his eyesight, Chris and Andrea peppered him with questions. Though he was still on the ventilator, he communicated by nodding his head yes or shaking his head no as they asked him questions.

Apparently, the questions were rattled off in succinct fashion because they did not know how long they would be able to talk to him.

"Can you hear us okay?"

"Yes," bobbed the little head.

"Are you in pain?"

"No," he wagged.

I don't know what all other questions they asked him, I forgot to find that piece of information out. I was so thrilled that he could hear and that he was not in pain that I didn't think of anything else that mattered right then. Hearing was one of those things that the neurosurgeon had said might be affected by the surgery. Knowing that Ryan could hear was a huge relief.

Chris explained to me that Ryan's ICP had risen to about 24, while all of this excitement took place. The doctors wanted the ICP to be below 20, but they were pleased with a 24, especially when it was compared to the reading that had been present throughout the previous week.

Even though Ryan was agitated about not being able to see, his pulse, and blood pressure remained stable during the initial awakening, so the doctors immediately decided to let him remain "awake." Actually, they gave him enough pain medication that it caused him to be sleepy, but they removed the sedative that caused him to be unconscious.

The doctors had been trying to keep Ryan with enough paralytic and sedative to keep him immobile and unconscious. They aimed for the point where he had enough paralytic and sedative to hold him in a suspended state, but not so much medication that his body and his mind shut down completely. When they had decided to remove the paralytic, they did not expect him to work his way out of sedation. The doctors and nurses had told us along the way that the ball was in Ryan's court. The better he tolerated something, the more they proceeded in that direction. The plan had been to reduce the sedative the middle of the next week and see how he responded, but when he fought past the sedative and woke up with the removal of the paralytic a hasty decision was made to see how he responded. Good ICP numbers, pulse rate, and blood pressure encouraged the doctors to let Ryan remain off the sedative.

As the sedative cleared from his system, it was obvious to everyone around him that Ryan was cognizant of who he was and where he was. This was a huge weight off everyone's shoulders because it indicated that mentally he was in good condition. Chris asked Ryan if he had a headache. Ryan shook his head "No," he was headache free. The fact that he did not have a headache was also a very good sign because it meant that the pressure inside his head was acceptable.

As the afternoon passed, a number of questions would arise by many, many people, questions, which did not then or now have answers. We all wondered the level at which Ryan would be able to function in a mental and a physical manner. We still did not know the level that Ryan would achieve, but for this afternoon we knew he was so vastly improved that we were all utterly amazed.

In less than twenty-four hours, Ryan had improved vastly, from a state of paralysis and unconsciousness, unable to tolerate even the slightest touch of someone's hand. On Friday, he reacted negatively if his body got outside a very specific temperature range. He was now awake, though groggy from the pain medication, and holding his own on all of his vital signs. The nurses cleaned the salve off Ryan's eyes and he and Chris watched the Arkansas Razorbacks game that evening. Though he still had a tube down his throat and he was on a significant amount of pain medication, Ryan was awake and aware of the game.

Incredibly, within a few hours of Ryan's awakening, the "Nation of Prayer Map" was completed as someone from Idaho signed the guestbook, completing the quest to have someone from each of the fifty states sign in saying they were praying for Ryan. By the time Ryan could see and was alert enough to understand the project, it was completed. I do not believe it was a coincidence that the map was completed and Ryan awoke within hours of each other. I fully believe that it was only because of the prayers of God's people that Ryan awakened at all. Within one week of starting the CaringBridge site, every state in the Union had a representative who had signed the guestbook assuring the family they were praying for Ryan.

I sat at my desk back in Centralia and I wept at the goodness of God. My dear little nephew, whom I had prayed over and had wept over, had not only survived, he was awake.

I was certain of one thing. Prayer had been an incredibly important part of Ryan's recovery to that point. My quest was to continue urging people to pray for Ryan's continued recovery. He was still not out of the woods entirely, but instead of being lost in the middle of the darkest heart of the woods, he was on the edge of the woods smiling and waving to all of those who had been praying for him. I knew he was a pretty tough kid, but I did not understand just how tough he really was. I went to bed that night in my own bed for the first time in a week. I went to sleep for the first time in a week with a peace that Ryan was awake. There was still a long way to go, but he was now on track for going forward. I had no idea, nor did any of the doctors, just how amazing his forward progress would be.

After I returned to Centralia, my involvement in Ryan's life took a different twist. I had been right by his bedside through the entire first week, but I could not stay there indefinitely. I had returned home and as such, I would spend many hours on the phone calling Little Rock to find out how Ryan was doing. Chris, Andrea, Nonna, Jenti, Laura and I all had cell phones, which were with the same company, and as such, we had free minutes to talk to each other. There would be times that I couldn't get anyone on the phone and in those times, I, like everyone else, would check the website to see what was happening. The first morning after I returned home, I prepared to go to church and preach. Early on that Sunday morning, I was unable to reach anyone by phone. Not to be deterred, I decided to check the website. On the website that morning, Chris was praising God for the power of prayer and the miracles that God had wrought in Ryan's life, which had culminated in Ryan awakening the day before.

My heart soared as I read the words. Not only was Ryan much improved, Chris was able to testify to the power of prayer. As I said earlier, we had been raised in church, but being able to speak outwardly in a fashion that glorifies God is something that I believe to be a learned art. It feels unnatural for most people when they start telling others how good God is; however, I believe it is essential that we learn to give praise to God when He blesses us. Jesus said even the rocks would cry out if we don't offer praises. To see that Chris had been able to put his thoughts into words was very moving. I knew God was working in Ryan's life and in the entire situation. It was just incredible to see that my little brother was openly able to express his gratitude to God for what He was doing in Ryan's life.

Chris had bought the movie *Cars* during one of our quick trips out to get supplies the previous week. He refused to open it until he and

Ryan could watch it together. Chris and I have pretty much the same philosophy about movies. Unless the movie has dramatically greater viewing pleasure on the big screen, it is more financially prudent to wait until it comes out on DVD and then purchase it to keep. Before being diagnosed, Ryan had known the movie was coming out on DVD and he had been looking forward to his dad purchasing it. While Ryan was in the coma, Chris had made sure to purchase a DVD of the movie. He wanted to be certain that when Ryan was able to watch the video, it would be there. While Ryan drifted in and out of sleep, Chris let the little guy know the movie was there when he was ready to watch it. Everyone caring for Ryan was very anxious for him to get to watch the movie. They had heard he really wanted to see the movie and they were pulling for him to be able to watch it very soon.

I am not sure why Ryan had touched the lives of the staff the way he did. They see children in and out of the hospital all of the time. Many of them are just as sick; some do not survive. I don't know if it was because of the family support that Ryan was getting, or if they just could sense he was a very special case, but the doctors and nurses were very involved in what was going on not only with Ryan but also with our family who was in the waiting room. We were told numerous times by the staff members that they were keeping up with Ryan's case through the CaringBridge site even on their days off. He had grabbed their hearts, and that grip would only continue to get tighter as time passed.

While I was preaching the morning sermon, Andrea made an update to the website. I was able to read the latest news as soon as the morning service was over. In the time that I was gone to church, the doctors had visited Ryan and determined that it was time to start trying to wean him off the ventilator. When someone has been on a ventilator for a while, the ventilator cannot be immediately stopped with the expectation that the body will begin to breathe on its own.

The procedure for removing the ventilator was to turn the level of assistance down gradually. The goal was to decrease the amount of assistance a little each day for about three days and by the end of the third day, the patient could be ventilator free. In Ryan's case, they were hoping to have him off the ventilator by Tuesday sometime. In addition, they had determined that the new altered respiratory therapy had been successful and Ryan's lungs were sounding clear. The cooling blanket had been completely removed from his bed. There would be no further need of it.

I could hardly believe the progress. Not only was he awake and aware of what was going on around him, they had already started making plans to get him off the ventilator. At least one of the tubes that was down Ryan's nose provided his food supply. He still had the ventilator tube down his throat, and still had IVs abounding. However, he was awake and trying to breath on his own. At the same time, he had stabilized to the point that the concern over his ICP and CPP had become secondary to the treatment of his lungs.

Overall, his level of care had begun to make a significant turn in the right direction. With the ICP and CPP finally holding stable, Ryan could receive care that was more comprehensive. The focus shifted from containing pressures to working on his lungs and beginning physical therapy on his left side. We had spent so many hours by his bedside with him in the "valley of the shadow of death" that just having him with stable cranial pressures was a blessing.

I talked to Nonna and Chris throughout the afternoon, at least a couple of times and each time I talked with them they were just vocally beaming. You could hear the joy in their voices. Fatigue had fallen by the wayside, at least for the time being. To be able to walk back to Ryan's room and see him awake made everyone a little livelier. It caused them to walk with a spring in their step. My biggest regret at the time was that I was not able to see him in this condition. Though I wished I could have seen him awake, I was still rejoicing long distance in the blessings that were being poured out on him.

Sunday ended as no other day had in quite some time. Ryan was alert, awake, and stable. Saturday had been the beginning of this phase, but Sunday was the first whole day, which found him in this condition. It allowed each person familiar with Ryan's case to go to bed with the hope that he was finally out of the woods and heading toward a rapid recovery. I don't believe at that point in time anyone could have anticipated the recovery Ryan would have. There really were no projections or predictions, just absolute revelry in his being awake and alert. The rest of his recovery was in the future and if we had learned anything to that point, it was that we did control the future. We consciously chose to live in the present and let the future take care of itself. The most pressing question for that night was whether Chris and Ryan would watch *Cars*.

As Monday morning dawned, I was back home and getting back into the routine. Some things did not change though, as always, I went straight to the CaringBridge site to see how the night before had gone.

I found that Chris had updated during the middle of the night. Ryan was having troubles resting and he had kept trying to get out of bed. They had given different types of medicine to help him rest, but something they tried to give him caused him to hallucinate. He kept reaching out into the air in an attempt to grab things that were not there. It was a little odd that Ryan was reaching for things that were not present, but medicine can play some very strange tricks on the mind. Years ago when our grandpa, Calvin, was suffering from cancer, the doctors gave him Tylenol with codeine for the pain. That caused him to see an elephant charging through the living room one day. After that, he put the medicine away and did not take it again because he did not like the hallucinations. The fact that Ryan was hallucinating was not a major concern, but it did bring a need to adjust his medications a little bit.

As I read the journal, I could sense that Chris was just elated by the progress. The level of ventilator assistance continued to be adjusted downward. The monitor for the ventilator contained color-coded lines. The nurses could tell by the color codes how many breaths Ryan initiated and how many the ventilator initiated. Through the night hours, he had continued to initiate more of his breaths and the ventilator initiated fewer and fewer.

Andrea was able to update the website mid-morning. I was so glad they were sticking to a good routine on updating since I had left. There was the early morning update that gave the previous night's summary, the mid-morning update that was done just before lunch, an afternoon update before people got off work, and then one more later in the evening, just before bedtime. As we had read the guestbook entries and had participated in numerous phone conversations, it was very clear that people wanted information as quickly as possible about Ryan.

When I read Andrea's mid-morning journal update, I noticed the talk had turned from ICP, CPP, critical, and dangerous to therapy and progress. I was in awe about the change in the language that everyone was using. When I talked with Chris, Andrea, or Nonna on the phone throughout the day, their voices seemed so much brighter. My heart was about to burst with gratitude to God. He had been right by our sides in the darkest of times and now we were able to rejoice in how gracious He was.

By Monday, it had been over one full week with the CaringBridge site up and running. There were people who told us along the way that they checked the site on their lunch hours and before leaving work because they did not have computers or internet access at home. On

Monday, those people who did not have internet access outside of work were finally finding out that Ryan was awake.

Two Sundays had passed since the whole ordeal started. That meant there had been two opportunities for prayer groups and churches to gather and pray for Ryan. The activity in the guestbook took off at an incredible pace. To read the guestbook caused an overwhelming sense of relief because of the knowledge there were so many people who were all over the country, and even around the world, holding Ryan up in prayer. The flood of kind words was unequaled as a source of comfort.

The difference from one Monday morning to the next cannot truly be understood I am afraid. One week prior to this day, Ryan was literally within seconds of death throughout the day. If the pressures had been uncontained at any point, he would have been unlikely to survive. God had been faithful and He had kept watchful care over Ryan throughout the darkest of hours. Now, one week later, Ryan was not only stabilized he was awake and alert and the doctors and nurses were moving him forward in his recovery at what seemed to be an amazing speed.

In the afternoon update, Andrea let me know she missed having me around to write the updates. I missed being there, but I pretty much knew I really was where I needed to be for the time being. My contact with Little Rock would remain continual, but further input from me into the journal would be some time away. That was fine though. I think that, while writing the journal entries, the author truly stopped and realized just how the situation was going at that time. I knew that in the worst of times I found it cathartic to write in the journal. I would realize just how overwhelming the entire situation could be, and it always helped to ground me and make me once again turn the day, the hour, or the minute back over to God.

During the day on Monday, Chris and a co-worker had gone in to check on Ryan. While they were in the room, Ryan moved his left leg. He was agitated and he wanted out of the bed. He squirmed around in the bed, and in doing so moved his left side. This was a huge emotional lift yet again. Though he had been "awake," he was still groggy much of the time due to the pain medication. This instance of movement on his left side was the most significant movement since he had awakened. This instance of movement gave us the assurance that Ryan was not paralyzed.

I switched from reading the updates to giving Chris a call. He explained to me that there had been a little problem in Ryan's breathing. He was not breathing enough on his own to continue with the ventilator settings that were currently being used. They had to increase the ventilator assistance, which was not good news. That meant they would not be able to remove it on Tuesday as we had been hoping. It also meant there was not going to be a definite timetable to remove the tube. Though it was a little discouraging, Ryan was so far ahead of where the doctors had expected him to be by this time; therefore, it was an acceptable compromise. When I had left on Saturday, the doctors were planning to try to cut back the sedatives and try to allow Ryan to start coming out of the coma on Tuesday or Wednesday. A setback with the ventilator was okay in my book when I considered he was not even supposed to be awake yet. I don't know that Chris agreed with me, but at least he was willing to be patient and he did not get really frustrated or distraught because of this step.

Chris had always been a dad who loved his kids, but when it came time for cleaning them or feeding them, it suddenly became Andrea's responsibility. I was impressed by how much of the responsibility he had shouldered during Ryan's hospital stay. He was spending every night in the room with Ryan and doing everything he could to help Ryan. That meant he spent a lot of one-on-one time with Ryan.

Many things happened in the wee hours during the days in the PICU, things to which Chris was the sole witness. As we spoke frequently, he would relate pertinent information to me and I would disperse it on the web as we agreed appropriate. We censored a lot of potentially discouraging information. Often the staff would alert Chris to possible complications or concerns. As it seemed counter-productive to alarm readers on speculation, we would withhold negative information until it was confirmed. It was a system that worked well, because often the concern ended up being unfounded. On the occasions when negative situations arose, we were cautious to share that information in words that were not overly pessimistic. We agreed to keep the website as positive as possible.

As one can imagine, this censoring of information placed a lot of stress on Chris. Many of the staff around him continued to watch Chris, waiting for him to lose his composure or have some sort of breakdown. When Chris never broke down, the staff became concerned that Chris was in denial about the severity of Ryan's condition. Chris assured them that he was fine; he realized the how dangerous Ryan's condition remained. Based on the ongoing conversations with Chris, I realized what was happening. He was not denying the crisis; he was trusting God.

The Results Are In

Before I entered the ministry, I worked as a chemist. I worked at an environmental testing lab full-time for about ten years, and then I worked part-time, as they needed my help for years after. It just so happened I was working on Tuesday, November 14, 2006. I remember it quite well, not because I wanted to remember working at the lab, but it was while I was at work the day really began to unfold. It became another day etched into my heart and my mind.

The day began well. I took my kids to school and then drove about thirty miles to the lab. I was supposed to have worked during the week I had spent in Little Rock, but I called Steve, my supervisor and told him I could not work that week. Work was uneventful for much of the morning. At lunch, I called Nonna to find out what the latest information was. She told me the doctors had gotten the pathology report back. Chris and Andrea had a 2:00 p.m. meeting with the oncology doctors to discuss the report and the course of treatment. I told her I would call her back about 2:30 p.m. to find out what the doctors had to say. The building I worked in was a metal building and so I had to go outside to use my cell phone. I remember it was a very cold, damp day. It made for a very miserable time standing outside to talk on the phone. Little did I know at that time how much the weather really represented the news we were about to receive.

I called Nonna several times to find out the results of the meeting, but it was a lengthy meeting and it had started late. About 3:30 p.m., I placed yet another call and found that Chris and Andrea had gotten back from their meeting. As they called some people, I talked with Nonna. My heart broke as I heard the news.

In tears, Nonna reported, "It is as bad as it can be. I don't know all of the details, but it is the most aggressive form of cancer and it is in the most advanced stage, a level four, the doctor said."

It would be a few weeks before I saw the pathology report firsthand, but when I did read it, the pathology report listed the tumor as an "Astrocytoma" under the general category heading. The specific type of tumor, within that category was listed as "Glioblastoma multiforme." "Category – 4", which turned out to be the most advanced level according to the rating scale used to describe cancer.

"I can't talk about it right now," Nonna wept. "I will talk to you later," and she hung up.

I stood there in a cold drizzle, stunned yet again. I had such high hopes that once Ryan got past the initial surgery, he would rapidly recover and get back to being a little boy again. I slowly walked back into the building, where the first person I saw was Steve. I must have been wearing the dismay openly on my face because he immediately wanted to know what was wrong.

I hesitated for fear of breaking into tears, and then I replied, "The pathology report is in. Ryan's cancer is the worst possible kind at the most advanced level."

I began to choke up and had to stop at that point. Steve responded, "I am so sorry, is there anything I can do to help? Do you need to leave? If you need to leave, don't worry about this place, we will get by without you."

"There is no reason to leave, there isn't anything I can do now but pray," I managed.

"Well, I will pray with you," Steve comforted.

The rest of the afternoon was a blur, but I made it through to the end. I got in the car and headed home. While I drove, I called Chris to talk with him for a bit about how he was doing after they had finished talking with the doctors.

"Hello," he woodenly answered.

"How are you all doing?" I tried to sound cheery, but in actuality didn't.

"We are getting by," he droned.

I could tell that I was going to have to carry the conversation. It was not an easy topic to broach, but I wanted to know the details of the meeting with the doctor. I engaged Chris in some small talk and finally I just asked him, "So what did the doctor have to say in the meeting. Mom told me it was really bad, but she didn't have any specifics other than it was level four."

With a sigh he began, "The doctor told us what type of tumor it was and how advanced it was. I asked him if they could tell what had caused the tumor to grow. He told us that it had probably been formed during Ryan's development in the womb. He believes that Ryan has had this thing his entire life. He speculated that some of the sinus headaches Ryan had been treated for his whole life could have actually been caused by the tumor rather than sinus problems.

"Typically, a tumor of this type, in that location would have caused seizures and alerted the doctors earlier that a problem was present. For some reason, Ryan never presented seizures and as such, the tumor had grown unabated and undetected his entire life."

"Unbelievable," I spouted.

Chris continued, "The oncologist told us they had designed a course of treatment. When Ryan is strong enough, he will start chemotherapy and radiation therapy simultaneously. He will have chemotherapy every day for forty-two straight days and he will have radiation therapy every Monday through Friday of that timeframe, for a total of thirty radiation treatments. The two treatments will then end at the same time."

"What happens if you decide not to make him take the treatments?" I questioned. It was my feeble attempt to find out if they were going to pursue the rigorous treatment. I wondered if they would want to put him through all of the pain of treatment or just take him home and make him as comfortable as possible for as long as possible.

Emphatically squelching any prospect of giving up, Chris retorted, "Well, the tumor will continue to grow and he will continually suffer from the pain and pressure he has dealt with to this point. However, it will get worse as time passes. We are going to pursue the course of treatment that the doctor suggests and pray for the best."

I must have touched a nerve with the last question because he told me he needed to go as quickly as the last exchange cleared his mouth. "I will talk with you later," were the last words out of his mouth, and then he was gone.

I couldn't blame him for being upset. He had gotten the report and later I found that the doctor had given him some scary statistics during that meeting. He received the information, but it was the same information Mames had come to the hospital with the day following Ryan's surgery. The very depressing information that Mames had found at that time was actually the information that dealt with the form and stage of cancer that Ryan actually did have. Since we knew what type and grade of cancer, we were able to rethink the information, but this time it wasn't speculation, it was reality.

The tumor was a type of cancer that typically strikes adults. The fact that it had attacked someone as young as Ryan was an anomaly. The statistics showed that if the entire tumor was removed, only 11% of the patients survived more than two years. Ryan's tumor had not been completely removed. The statistics also showed that even if the tumor was removed completely and chemotherapy and radiation were performed, there was a high likelihood that the cancer would return. The one statement that hit me the hardest was the statement that said there had been no improvements in the treatment for this type of cancer in the past 25 years.

I called Chris again after I got home and had dinner. I wanted to give him a little space, but I still had questions I wanted answered. As can be imagined, he was very downhearted. I engaged in a little small talk once again, but I had to know the answer to one question especially, so I finally ventured to ask that question. "How much time do the doctors say that Ryan has left?"

He paused for a moment and then began. "The doctors here at ACH won't give a prognosis involving a timetable. They are very fact oriented. If a child is alive, they do not speculate on how long that child will live. They do their best to give the child the longest, most productive life that child can expect to have. They will treat Ryan as long as there is hope, and in their opinion, as long as he is alive there is hope. The oncologist told me, 'We do not give a prognosis based on statistics, because children are not statistics.'"

I was very impressed by the way the doctors were moving forward in Ryan's care, but I did not know how much expertise ACH had in pediatric oncology. I asked Chris if they had considered transferring Ryan to St. Jude Hospital, in Memphis, Tennessee. St. Jude was a pediatric cancer research hospital. Chris and I had both been in BETA club in high school and our group raised money for St. Jude every year. They were an outstanding hospital, very cutting edge when it came to treatment options.

"Actually, the oncologist at ACH called St. Jude to see if they could do anything different for Ryan. The head oncologist recently left St. Jude to take a job in Arizona. The oncologist at ACH found that the rest of the staff at St. Jude was in complete agreement with the course of treatment prescribed by ACH. The big difference is ACH has a rehabilitation ward and St. Jude does not."

Chris expounded on the rehabilitation. "The doctors' panel with oncology, neurology, and therapy all discussed Ryan this morning before they talked with us. The plan is to keep Ryan in the hospital and aggressively pursue occupational, speech, and physical therapies. They want the whole package to benefit as much as possible and if he goes to St. Jude, they will only pursue the oncology perspective. Andrea and I agreed we had trusted ACH this far and we were going to stay the course with them. They have saved his life; we trust them to help make the right decisions from here forward."

We conversed for a bit longer, but it was clear the decisions were set in stone. ACH would be the place Ryan was treated and everyone got on board with that decision very quickly. Chris and Andrea were correct in their assessment. There was no need to change hospitals at that point, they had already saved his life, and all the staff had a vested interest in helping Ryan get better.

Shortly after I got off the phone with Chris, Nonna called me and asked me to call and check on Poppa. She said when she had talked with him he was pretty shaken. I heard from Jenti also, and she was very upset. She had been with dad shortly after we had gotten the original report. She said he had just gone white with the news. He was staying at home by himself and they were concerned about how he was. Therefore, I called to talk with him for a while.

When I was talking with Poppa, he assured me he was doing okay. He had been shaken by the news, but he believed that Ryan had come through too much for God just to let him be taken so quickly by the cancer. Poppa told me he believed Ryan was going to be a miracle for us to be able to tell others about how good God is. I do not think any more prophetic words have ever been spoken.

With the events that had happened throughout the day, we did have some good news, Ryan was off the ventilator and he was able to speak. Though there had been a small setback earlier, he began to make such rapid progress that he made up the difference and the ventilator was removed on the original schedule. He was beginning to show good signs of improvement, but we really did not know what that might mean considering the pathology report. We did know he had to be physically stronger before the cancer could be treated.

We had committed Ryan's care to God and that was where it would stay. Whatever came, we had all agreed we would trust God to give us the grace to see us through it. After I heard the pathology results, I considered making a return trip to Little Rock. However, with the Thanksgiving holiday rapidly approaching, I decided I would not make the trip to Little Rock at that time. Laura and I discussed the situation and decided if Ryan were still in the hospital at Thanksgiving, we would go to Little Rock as a family to spend the holiday.

My kids were longing to see Ryan. They had been without their dad for over a week and had read the journal. They had all posted words of encouragement on the guestbook, and they had been praying for him the entire time. They would hear bits and pieces as Laura and I would talk after a phone call sometimes, but we felt it best not to overload them with the dismal statistics about the cancer Ryan had. We did our best to help them deal with their feelings, and we answered all of their questions as honestly as we could. They really wanted to go to Little Rock and to Ryan, but there just was not any way we could go before Thanksgiving. They accepted the plan without much complaint. They just wanted to see Ryan for themselves.

After the ventilator tube was removed, one of the first things that Ryan wanted to do was watch *Cars* with his dad. What a blessedly simple request, and it had been a terribly long time in coming to pass. On that night, after receiving such a horrible diagnosis, Chris shared the evening with his baby boy, just the two of them watching the movie that had been the dream of a child to see.

Andrea made a journal update on Wednesday morning that made me laugh. I had to call Chris and check the story out firsthand.

Chris answered the phone with an audibly cheerier tone, "Good morning."

"Tell me the whole story about what Andrea mentioned on the site this morning," I prodded.

He began to laugh aloud, and when he regained his composure, he began, "As quickly as Ryan had the tube removed, he began to try to talk. He was hoarse and he couldn't speak above a whisper, but he was once again able to communicate with words. He began to ask, of all things, about what was happening at his school. He said he missed Mrs. Kennemer and his classmates. He was ready to return to school right then. Shortly after lunch, he took a nap and when he awoke, he tried to get out of bed. He was going to dress himself and go to school. The nurse had a tough time convincing him that he was not supposed to get out of bed. The nurse had an even tougher time convincing Ryan that he did not have to school that day. Ryan argued with the nurse for quite a while, but it made him tired, so he lay down for another nap. While he was asleep, I left the room for a bit. When I returned, the nurse was turning the room upside down looking for something. Ryan was craning his neck giving advice about where IT could be. I couldn't help but crack up laughing when the nurse said, 'Ryan told me he had homework in his backpack. He asked me to get his papers out so he can work on them. I have looked everywhere, but I can't seem to find his backpack.' The nurse thought I had finally lost my mind when I started laughing. They keep waiting for me to crack you know. The nurse asked me if I was all right. 'More alright than you know,' I answered. 'Ryan does not have any homework, and there is no backpack. He was just a little confused, but he was mentally sharp enough to convince you he did. I think my little boy is going to be just fine,'" and, concluding his account, Chris began to roar with laughter once again. I had a good chuckle as well about the whole story.

Having read the CaringBridge guestbook entries from Mrs. Kennemer, I could see why Ryan was so fond of her. She was extremely compassionate and she cared deeply about each and every one of her students. I had been surprised to find out Ryan was not her first student to battle cancer. Actually, she had another student in her class, a friend of Ryan's, who had undergone many of the same types of treatments that Ryan was to undergo. He had a different form of cancer, but the treatment was similar. Several people had indicated they would read the journal and if I had written the entry, they usually cried. They said they would then read the guestbook with an entry from Mrs. Kennemer, they cried some more. The compassion and the love Mrs. Kennemer had poured out on her class had touched them so deeply that they all loved school. They loved to learn. They enjoyed school. Ryan was no exception and he missed school.

The second thing Ryan wanted addressed after the ventilator was gone was food. He had been hungry the night he had flown to Little Rock. Twelve days into his treatment and he still had not had any solid food. On Wednesday, he was finally strong enough to have solid food. Chris let me know they were going to perform another CT scan and following the CT scan he had promised to get Ryan something solid to eat.

A CT scan was going to be done because the ICP had started to creep higher once again. The neurosurgeon who had performed the surgery was concerned about the pressure. When Ryan had been struggling against the high ICP previously, the doctor had talked about putting in a permanent shunt inside of Ryan's head to aid in draining fluid. The severe nature of his condition caused the doctor to avoid this procedure as long as possible. Since Ryan was now awake and getting stronger, the doctor wanted to see what was happening inside of Ryan's skull and determine if fluid was still accumulating. The CT scan showed there was indeed a pooling of fluid. Based on the CT results, the doctor decided it would be best to insert a permanent shunt inside Ryan's head. He did not wish to rush into the procedure, so he discussed the situation with Chris and Andrea and determined the first part of the next week they would take Ryan back into surgery and insert the shunt.

The news of the shunt insertion was not the best news for us to hear, but it was not nearly as traumatic as it would have been in those early days of Ryan's recovery. One thing the doctor indicated was he had hesitated to insert the shunt initially because he did not know if Ryan was strong enough to survive the procedure. Following the CT scan, the doctor was confident Ryan was strong enough to have the procedure done, and he was confident it would help to alleviate the spiking in the ICP.

One day removed from the ventilator, Ryan was visited by the physical therapy staff. They helped him sit up in bed, the first time he had sat up in nearly two weeks. During the initial visit by the therapist, Ryan was able to move his left leg, left foot, and left arm. The movement was not very strong; however, he did have the ability to move them under his own strength. This meant he might have diminished ability on that side, but he was not going to be paralyzed.

And so, a new phase had begun. Ryan was awake, eating, and talking. He was able to sit up now, though it was limited. With his return to sitting up, Ryan was able to get into a wheelchair for the first time. Once in the wheelchair, he was able to go anywhere in the hospital. After he had been awake for just four days, he was being wheeled around the hospital, checking out all of the sights.

The wheelchair was a special type of chair. Ryan could be buckled into the chair so he did not slip out. It was a child sized wheelchair and it reclined. When Ryan got tired, all he had to do was ask his "driver" to lean the seat back a little bit and he would drop off to sleep. The wheelchair became one very good way to motivate Ryan to do the things he needed to do. He really got tired of being in his bed and loved to spend time sitting in his wheelchair. As there was a strong possibility Ryan could be in a wheelchair for the rest of his life, Chris and Andrea used it as a positive reinforcement rather than making it seem negative in any fashion. If Ryan took his medicines and breathing treatments as he was supposed to, then he was able to get into his wheelchair.

Once Ryan was able to get into a wheelchair, the doctors decided he was strong enough to be in a regular room. So, on Thursday evening, less than one week after he awoke, Ryan was moved out of the PICU.

I happened to call Nonna, not knowing Ryan was to be moved. We talked while she sat in Ryan's room with him. Chris and Andrea were moving Ryan's belongings while Nonna and I talked.

"So how are things?" I asked.

With a chuckle, Nonna said, "Well, it looks like the circus is leaving town."

"Huh?" I quizzically muttered.

She continued, "We are moving to a regular room on the fourth floor. You saw how many stuffed animals and balloons Ryan had been given. Well, since you left, he has received probably twice that many more. To move all of his stuff from this room to the new room, Chris and Andrea are using those wagons that are all around the hospital. They come in with three wagons at a time and fill each of them to the top. Chris tows two wagons at a time to the new room and Andrea falls in line behind him with the third wagonload. With all of those animals in the wagons, it looks just like a circus train leaving town."

We talked for a few more minutes, about how everything was going at the hospital. It was very exciting to hear Ryan had progressed to the point he could be out of the PICU finally. Ryan had been in the PICU since he had entered the hospital. This was the first time he had moved and it was the first night he would spend without the staff being within a few feet of his bed. When the doctors made the determination he was strong enough to leave the PICU it was yet another incredible blessing to all of us.

As I talked with Nonna that evening, she told me of some secret plans that were going to be executed the next day. I had to smile when she told me what was going to happen. It was with much anticipation that I looked forward to hearing how events of the next day would unfold. Little did I know just how emotional the next day would be for me as well.

On Friday morning, the first morning with Ryan being away from the PICU, Laura, my wife, had called to talk to Chris about how Ryan was doing after his move. During the conversation, Chris told her there was someone there that wanted to talk to her. She expected it to be Andrea, but suddenly there was Ryan on the other end of the line.

"I love you, Aunt Laura," she heard and then Ryan handed the phone back to his dad.

Laura called me to tell me she had gotten to talk to Ryan. I immediately called back to see if I could talk to him for a few minutes.

"Hi, Uncle Tim," came a tiny little weak voice. Chris had seen my name on the caller ID and had given the phone to Ryan to answer.

"It sure is great to hear your voice. How are you feeling?" I brokenly uttered.

"I am doing fine. Thank you for coming to see me while I was in the hospital. I have to go now; I have to rest my voice. I love you."

"I will talk to you later." I hung up and sat at the desk crying tears of joy. This was the first time I had gotten to hear him since the night I had gotten to Little Rock. He sounded so small and frail. He could not speak very loud because of the tube that had been down his throat and it was difficult to understand his words because they were so soft. Though his voice was quiet, the message was very loud and clear.

Ryan probably would have talked a little longer, but Chris cut him off. Ryan needed to save his voice for the special surprise. The secret plans that Nonna had told me about the night before were about to be set in motion and those plans required Ryan to talk. I completely understood.

November 16, was Mrs. Kennemer's birthday. Chris and Andrea had worked it out with the school for Ryan to call her at 2:00 p.m. to wish her a Happy Birthday. She had not been able to see him since he had awakened from his long sleep, so they decided to surprise her for her birthday.

The guestbook on the CaringBridge site was a very special place through which we could escape from reality. We spent hours reading the words of encouragement. Some people wrote their prayers for our family out on the guestbook pages. Those words of encouragement carried us through many difficult stretches. As it is a very personal document, one into which people around the world have poured their hearts, I would feel odd about publishing their words without getting everyone's permission. However, in this instance, I am going to include a very special entry that was made in the guestbook. It was from Mrs. Kennemer. She made the entry Friday night after an eventful birthday. It expressed the emotion of the day more eloquently than I ever could.

FRIDAY, NOVEMBER 17, 2006 09:41 PM, CST

Dear Ryan, Let me see...there are no words to describe how I felt the moment I heard your precious voice. I will never ever forget the most wonderful birthday present that I have ever received. Sweetheart, I am not sure if you know just how important it was for me to be able to talk with you today. You brought so many smiles and tears today, and just to let you know, those tears were of joy. I promise to try to keep them under control tomorrow while I am with you, but today, they flowed freely and not just while I was listening to you, but for the rest of the day. It was a true blessing, and I have thanked the good Lord all day ... Ms. Sheri called me to the office for a phone call. I never receive phone calls during the day; so, she had to repeat what she had said. This time it sunk in quickly. You would be amazed at how fast I ran to the office. Yes, believe me when I say "RAN." I know that I impressed every one I passed. I was on a mission and I got there in record time. Thank you Sweetie for making me so happy. Having you

*there talking to me today has given me so much strength.
You are such a Go Getter. You stay strong for all of us and
remember that my faith in you is still there and getting
stronger each day. Oh, the smiles. You made all of your
friends so happy. They were cheering you on. You have
the best cheering squad. I cannot wait until tomorrow. I
am so thankful I will get to see you and talk with you
without the phone being in between each of us. Thanks,
Dad, for giving us the update on the Happy Meal and the
ice cream ... Sleep tight, Kiddo, and again, thank you for
my wonderful birthday present. It will always have a
special place in my heart. Love you forever, Mrs.
Kennemer*

It was now two weeks to the day since Ryan had been diagnosed
with a mass in his head. The previous Friday, I had been in Little Rock
watching over him as he slept. Ryan's pressures were still somewhat
problematic, but far less trouble than one week earlier. So much had
changed during the second week. People had continued to bombard
Heaven with prayers for Ryan. I believe we could see the hand of God
working through each day to restore Ryan's body. My biggest regret
was I was not there to witness it firsthand. I had to be contented with
talking to the family by phone and reading the journal entries. It hadn't
hurt to hear his soft little voice either.

As it was once again Friday, Nurse Valerie came back on duty.
Since Ryan was no longer in the PICU, Nurse Valerie was not Ryan's
nurse. However, when she reported to work and found out Ryan had
been moved, she made it a point to visit the fourth floor and see Ryan
during her break. She was astounded when she saw him. It had been a
week since her last experience with him. When she saw him this time,
he was sitting in his wheelchair. He had colored a picture for her. It
had been an exceptionally upbeat day and Chris published updated
information on the site about the "Nation of Prayer Map." In that first
two-week period, word had spread and Ryan had people praying for him
in all fifty states and in twenty-five nations around the world. It was
obvious when one looked at the progress he had made that the power of
prayer had played a huge role in his recovery.

It was time for the weekend again. The number of visitors had
dropped off through the week, but many people visited over the
weekend. Ashtyn was taken back to Little Rock and Mrs. Kennemer
was able to visit that weekend. Ashtyn was beginning a week of school

break and she would be able to stay in Little Rock until after Thanksgiving. The plans were tentatively set that she would stay at the RMH with Andrea and Nonna.

Gratitude was overwhelming Chris and Andrea's hearts. Ryan was so much better; he wanted to spend a lot of time sitting up coloring. When Ashtyn arrived in Little Rock on Saturday, they got to sit side by side and color. That must have been a beautiful sight. The bond between the two of them is so strong that one might wonder if they were twins. It was very difficult on Ashtyn to see her little brother in such terrible shape when she had gone home, but now that he was awake and able to sit up they had a very good chance to spend time together.

When I talked to anyone in Little Rock, it was getting very apparent everyone was getting restless. When Ryan had gone into the hospital, we had discussed the upcoming Thanksgiving holiday. We had decided we would need to wait and see how Ryan was doing before any plans were made concerning the holiday. As the days and weeks had passed, it became apparent Ryan would be in the hospital on Thanksgiving. We talked about plans for the holiday. Everyone really wanted all of us to be together for Thanksgiving. We always spent the holidays together if possible. This year held a special significance, because we truly had so much for which to be thankful.

We talked with Poppa and he planned to make the trip back to Little Rock for the holiday, as did Jenti, Steve, and their boys. Laura searched around the web and found a hotel we could stay at which was closer to the hospital than the one in which we had previously stayed. They had a slightly higher rate, but they also had much larger rooms. We all reserved rooms at that hotel, so we could be in the same building. We worked out what we wanted to have to eat for Thanksgiving and we worked on planning a birthday party for Ashtyn. Her birthday was the day before Thanksgiving Day, so a party was in order for that as well.

Rather than counting the hours or minutes, we had finally arrived at the place we could count the days. The days that Ryan had been out of a coma, the days until Thanksgiving, the days until he had the shunt inserted into his head. We stopped living our lives from hour to hour and started living day to day, which was quite a move from the way we had been living for the previous two weeks. I believe everyone was in one accord that we were thrilled with the progress Ryan had made and we all looked forward to the holidays that were rapidly approaching.

Physical therapy (PT) and occupational therapy (OT) went hand in hand with each other. The therapists did an incredible job of coming up with the activities that worked the proper muscle groups without getting tiresome. Prior to the insertion of the shunt, the therapists worked on stretching Ryan's muscles. They devised games to help stretch his muscles, but the therapists did not want to be overly ambitious with therapy with the ICP/CPP still fluctuating. The plan was to become more extensive with his therapy after the shunt was inserted and the ICP regulated. As the procedure to insert the shunt drew near, Chris and Andrea became a little more apprehensive. They had relished the days that had been passing with Ryan laughing and coloring, playing games and eating everything in sight. They did not like the idea of him going back into surgery, but they knew it was necessary.

The shunt was to be placed on the left side of Ryan's skull, the side opposite the tumor. The doctors wanted to make certain the shunt would not interfere with any other treatments Ryan would be having. Everything about the surgery to place the shunt was well designed before it was ever undertaken. The placement of the shunt itself was critical for the drainage to work as it should. The CT scan that had been done the previous week gave the doctors the information as to where the shunt had to be placed. The doctor did not need an MRI to place the shunt at this time. At the time of his surgery, Ryan's brain was so malformed because of swelling, tumor, and fluid that they needed the extra detail of an MRI to find the "landmarks" that let them know about the regions of Ryan's brain. As the weeks passed, the swelling had reduced and the fluid level had dropped. A CT scan was sufficient to direct the shunt placement. The drain which had been placed in Ryan's head on the day of the surgery, had been removed prior to his leaving the PICU. Without that, the ICP/CPP could not be monitored numerically. Though he had made it for days without a drain, the doctors did not want to risk possible future complications, thus they were insistent a permanent internal drain needed to be in place.

The day of the procedure dawned and preparations to take Ryan to surgery were completed early. He went to surgery and within a few tedious hours, Ryan was back in his room. By early afternoon, I talked with Nonna and found out Ryan's procedure was completed. He was back in recovery and headed very shortly to his room. He had finished yet another step in his recovery. During the drain insertion process, the sutures from the first surgery were removed. Ryan returned to his room with an internal drain that could be seen just below the surface of his skin and a small incision where the drain had been inserted. His scar was healing nicely and he was down to one IV. All other monitors, pumps, tubes, and drains had been removed. He was well on his way to mobility.

Ryan had the shunt inserted the Tuesday prior to Thanksgiving Day. The plan had been to perform an MRI the day after Thanksgiving to check the progress inside of Ryan's head. The doctors decided rather than intrude on the holiday gathering, they would perform the MRI on Wednesday before Thanksgiving. I was pleased they had decided to change the date of the MRI. It took several hours for Ryan to undergo the MRI and wake from the sedative they gave him to keep him still during the procedure. By the test being moved to the day we were all traveling to Little Rock, we would not have to have our time together interrupted by the procedure.

As I spoke on the phone that evening with Nonna and Chris, it was obvious they were relieved the shunt insertion was completed. They were now very excited about everyone gathering for Thanksgiving. We were all leaving our respective homes at different times on Wednesday, and our hope was to meet in Little Rock in the early afternoon, just in time for a birthday party for Ashtyn. I was extremely excited to be going back to Little Rock. I had not seen Ryan since the day I left him, unconscious in the PICU. He had made huge strides in his recovery, so I had been told. I was anxious to see for myself what God had done in the life of this amazing child. I spent a restless night that night in anticipation of the journey I would make the next day. This time though it was a good restlessness. I was going to witness firsthand the wonders of God and I was excited.

Giving Thanks

The day before Thanksgiving Day, we left home early and headed for Little Rock. While we were on the road, the doctors proceeded with the MRI and all of the other tests they wanted to check before the holiday weekend. As we traveled and the testing was completed, the decision was made to move Ryan to the rehabilitation ward on the fifth floor. Ryan had been on the fourth floor, which was the neurology ward. He was to be moved to the rehab ward so he could begin therapy that was more intensive. He had been visited by the therapists while he was on the fourth floor, but the move to the fifth floor indicated it was time to get serious about getting him up and about as much as possible. The doctors and therapists still did not have a clear indication as to what level his physical therapy would help him achieve, but they had decided to help him fulfill whatever potential was still within his little body.

In the days leading up to our trip to Little Rock, we became familiar with another child in the hospital. Her name was Cassie and while we were very excited about how Ryan was progressing, Cassie's prognosis was not so good. Her parents were staying in the RMH and Nonna and Andrea had gotten to know them. While we were on the way to Little Rock, Cassie passed away. Sadly, she was not the only child to pass away during Ryan's stay in the hospital. Every time we found out about a child who did not survive it just further touched our hearts that God had blessed us by letting Ryan stay around for a while longer. We all had come to realize how precious life was and we had decided to make the most of each day.

When we arrived at the hospital, it was early evening/late afternoon. We found Ryan in the room we had been told he would be in and when we walked in the whole room just lit up with Ryan's smile. He was sitting up in bed coloring a picture and he just glowed with excitement about seeing his cousins. Within just a short time, everyone else got to the hospital. It was party time as we began the holiday gathering with Ashtyn's birthday party. We all gathered in a section of the cafeteria and had the food that had been prepared for us. Aunt Lisa had prepared a cooler full of fried chicken. It had been tightly packed and was still slightly warm when it arrived. Jenti's father-in-law had smoked a turkey for us and trimmings of all types had been added to the bounty. I was a bit saddened when I found out Jenti and Steve's boys had stayed in Missouri with their other set of grandparents. When Jenti and Steve had gone to get the turkey, they had arranged for the boys to stay there as they were not sure how they would handle being in the hospital for the long weekend.

As we began to eat our meal, I sat down at the end of the table and witnessed a very funny battle of wills transpire. I had to stifle a laugh as I watched it unfold.

Jenti had filled a plate with food for Ryan and he began to eat. She filled her plate and sat down beside him. She had different food on her plate than he had.

"What else is there to eat?" he questioned Jenti.

"I don't know what all is up there on that table," she answered. "If you clean up your plate, I will take you over there and let you pick out anything you want to eat."

She had put two chicken legs and a few other items on Ryan's plate and he was eating one of the legs while they talked. Jenti turned her back to Ryan for a minute and talked to someone on the other side of the table. While she wasn't looking, Ryan took all the food off his plate and put it on her plate.

"Jenti, can we go see what's on the food table now?" he coyly queried.

As Jenti turned to respond, she realized his food was on her plate. "I told you I would take you over there when you ate all of your food, you didn't eat it you put it on my plate."

Ryan glanced over at me and smiled big and bright. "That's not what you told me Jenti. You said when my plate was clean you would take me to see what else was on that food table."

Mouth agape, voice unheard, Jenti started to protest, but she knew she had been outsmarted, she wheeled him to the food table and didn't bother trying to argue with him.

Ryan ate all of the food he wanted and then asked Jenti to lean his wheelchair back. After a brief fumbling attempt by Jenti, he leaned back and took a nap while everyone else sat and visited. After he had a nice nap, we went back to his room only to find he was going to be moved to yet another room. This time there were several extra people to help move things, so it went much quicker. We loaded wagons full of Ryan's stuff and took pictures off the walls. Nonna was correct. When Ryan changed rooms, it appeared as if the circus was leaving town.

As we moved Ryan into his new room, we found out the playroom on the fifth floor was just a few doors down the hall. The playroom had a TV with DVD player, video game systems, plus toys and games of every kind. Ryan thought it was a great room to visit with all of his cousins. The kids spent time in the playroom while we worked on getting Ryan's belongings into his room.

Throughout the afternoon and evening, Ryan would get tired and he would lay his little head down and doze off. After he had slept for a while, he would wake up and be back in the action. He wanted to stay in the wheelchair a lot more, but he could not stay in it full time because it caused swelling in his feet and legs. He was not very happy about having to get back in bed, but he accepted it finally. He, my daughters Jessica and Rebekah, and Ashtyn all colored pictures while Ryan was in bed. They did not want to leave his side unless they were forced to for some reason. Joshua, my son, spent a lot of time in the playroom. I figured it was because of the video game system, but I found out why a little later in the weekend.

My kids were relieved to see Ryan when we got to Little Rock. They had not seen him at any point during this whole event. They had either read about or heard everything they knew about his condition, but they had not witnessed anything firsthand. Now they could see him for themselves, it helped them to process everything they had been hearing.

It had been a long day for everyone involved and when it came time for visiting hours to end, we were pretty much all ready to head back to our hotel. The next day was Thanksgiving and we were overwhelmed with gratitude that we could all be together. It would not be the typical holiday, but we were all together and for that, we were extremely thankful.

On Thanksgiving Day, before we got to the hospital, Chris spoke with the neurosurgeon about the results of Ryan's MRI. The swelling was diminishing and the fluid was draining properly, thanks to the recently implanted shunt. The hemisphere line, the line that ran down the middle of the brain, separating the two halves, had been severely arced in the MRI on November 4. With the tumor removed, the line was straightening out, as there was once again space inside of Ryan's head. These were extremely good things to hear, especially from the neurological perspective. As the doctor prepared to leave Ryan's room after the consultation, he held up his hand to have Ryan "give him five." The doctor was shocked to see Ryan use his left hand to "give five" to the doctor. He was a plainspoken man and he told Chris he was amazed Ryan had the muscle control that allowed him to do that. The doctor told Chris he really had not ever expected Ryan to develop the motor abilities to do something like that with his left hand again, and the fact that he could do it that soon after the surgery was truly miraculous.

Chris was all aglow as we got to the hospital and he was able to share the encounter with us. That consultation set the tone for the whole day.

Thanksgiving Day is not all about food or football. It is not about Christmas sales or even about family gatherings. Those things are all part of how we celebrate. Thanksgiving Day is about being thankful for what the Lord has done for us. When the pilgrims celebrated, it was not because there would be a big sale the next day, it was because they were thankful they had survived. They were alive and they were thankful for that. Ryan was alive; we were all together there in the hospital, and for that, we were truly thankful.

Throughout the day, the kids would go back and forth to the playroom. Ryan was taken to the playroom for intervals, but when he tired, he returned to his room to rest. It was too noisy for even him to rest in the playroom. While Ryan rested, the other kids played. The hospital's rule was that all kids had to have an adult watching over them. Steve and Joshua spent a lot of time in the playroom, so that rule was obeyed. I walked past the room several times throughout the day and I saw different people playing the video game system that was in the room. I assumed Joshua was staying in the room to play the video game. I was mistaken.

There were two kids in the playroom that did not seem to have anyone watching them, which was against the rules. As the day passed, we found out more and more about those kids.

They were two, one boy and one girl, of three siblings. The third sibling, another girl, was in the burn ward of the hospital in serious condition. They said their mother had died. We could only assume that whatever had happened to place these three kids in the hospital was how their mother had passed away. Their father was working and they had a cousin that was "keeping an eye on them." We figured out the young man who was glued to the video game system most of the day was the person who was "in charge" of them, though he was not involved with them at all. Joshua always carried a deck of cards with him, as he loved to play all kinds of card games. He sat down with the little girl, and played a game with her. She beat him of course. It was odd, but he spent hours playing cards with that little girl. Later that evening I found out that he hadn't played the video game system at all.

"Can you pick up a deck of cards for me the next time you go to the store?" he requested.

"You have a deck of cards don't you?" I retorted.

"Not anymore. I let my new little friend have them," he reasoned.

"Oh, okay. Any particular reason?" I wondered aloud.

"She did not have any of her own. I felt sorry for her. She said that her mom had died. I didn't know what else to say, but she seemed to enjoy playing cards so I let her keep them," he explained.

We ended up eating in the cafeteria on Thanksgiving Day. We snacked on leftovers throughout the day and ate our "big family meal" in shifts in the cafeteria. My wife thoroughly enjoyed the food, but I missed having Nonna's home cooking. For the first time in my life, I can honestly say I did not eat too much at the Thanksgiving "feast."

The day was incredible to experience. As I walked the halls of the hospital, again I realized God had performed a mighty miracle in Ryan's life. Actually, I realized God was continually performing a miracle in our lives by allowing us to have Ryan with us.

I watched throughout the day as Chris interacted with Ryan. I was continually amazed at how much compassion he had with Ryan and how he helped Ryan in any way Ryan needed him. I made mental notes the whole day long as I was going to see if Chris wanted me to update the journal after I got back to the hotel. Before visiting hours ended, Chris talked with me about it and asked me if I would write a journal update. I asked him what he wanted it to say and he told me to write what I felt like I should write. He wanted the emotion and the thankfulness of all we had experienced to show through and he did not think he could do it justice. I smiled and told him I would take care of it.

I went back to the hotel and I prayed about how I should write this entry. Unbeknownst to anyone except Laura and one other prayer partner, I had been struggling a lot with the situation over the previous week or so. I did not know how I should feel or how I should pray. I wanted God to touch Ryan, but I did not feel as if He was going to do what I wanted Him to do. Then, one day I heard from God. It was a near audible voice, but not quite. I had the distinct impression that God was revealing what He wanted me to grasp. I felt I needed to share my struggles in the Thanksgiving Day journal update. As I poured my heart into the journal entry that night, I was able to share more than I had shared about my struggles and what I had learned through them.

THURSDAY, NOVEMBER 23, 2006 09:42 PM, CST
Uncle Tim here.
Chris asked me to do the final update for this
Thanksgiving Day, so I said I would. Grab a Kleenex and
read on if you want a lump in your throat.

One thing I have come to realize through the situation with this is that there are more questions in life than there are answers. If one gets caught up in asking questions, they often fail to hear the answers that are provided. It doesn't really do very much good to ask all of the questions in the world, especially if you aren't really trying to hear the answers.

I know there have been so many encouraging notes and comments, prayers and petitions on behalf of our family. I also know there have been many out there who have wondered why this type of thing happens, especially to someone like Ryan. Life is full of these questions, and often we cannot find the answers. I have decided rather than asking these questions I cannot get answers for, I would try to share the beauty of what God has been doing for us through this time.

When I heard the diagnosis, the results of the pathology report, I started trying to get answers from the internet about what the doctors told the family. Talk about discouraging. I started praying for a miracle, but I just did not have the assurance God was going to heal Ryan. I believe God is fully capable of miraculously healing Ryan, but I did not have a peace about the reality of God healing Ryan. I continued to pray and intercede on Ryan's behalf. About Friday of last week, I had a clear message I believe was from God. It was as if He were sitting right next to me while I was praying. I was really down, because I still did not believe Ryan was going to be physically healed, or at least not the way I was thinking. It was at that point in time, when I was feeling so low, I felt that God spoke to me and said, "I haven't told you what I am going to do yet. Do not be discouraged, just wait, and see." Immediately, my attitude changed, my heart lightened and my whole outlook on the situation has changed.

Today is Thanksgiving; hopefully you realized that before now. As we sat in Ryan's hospital room today, I felt so blessed to be with my family. We were missing a few members who would have been at Mom's house if we had been there. Li'l Steve, Devonta, Shannon, Lisa, Jason, Brittney, Jake and Skeeter, you were all missed. At Nonna's house, you actually never know who might show up on a holiday like today. However, as we sat in the hospital room, ate in the hospital cafeteria, and had leftovers from yesterday, I really know that I understand what being thankful is all about more than ever before.

About 10 days ago, I had to leave and go home. As Laura and I drove away from Little Rock, Ryan was still in a state of paralysis and completely sedated. I had not seen his eyes open since a little while after the surgery which saved his life the week before. About 2 1/2 hours after we left and headed home, I got a call on my cell phone and I was told Ryan had awakened. I was shocked. When I had left they were talking about trying to bring him out of that state toward the first part of the following week, but instead they had started adjusting his meds and he woke up within a couple of hours. I wanted to turn around and go back, but I did not really think we could do that and still get home at a decent time, so we went on home.

Through the following week, I kept calling the hospital and talking to my mom and my brother and my sister-in-law, and then last Friday, I was able to hear Ryan's weak little voice on the phone. Guess which day that was, you guessed it, that was the day I felt I had heard from God that He hadn't told me what He was going to do. I really do not remember which voice I heard first, God's or Ryan's.

We came to Little Rock to share Thanksgiving with the family, and we have to leave in the morning (after I take Mom Christmas shopping). Tonight Ryan did not want to do his breathing treatment. Chris had to get tough with him (he took Ryan's coloring book and colors until Ryan agreed to do his treatment). Ryan did his treatment and Chris gave his colors back.

It was such a blessing to see a battle of wills between father and son and realize this was the same battle I was fighting with my Father. I thought I had it all figured out, that I would be able to be strong for the rest of my family, as we had to deal with an un-inviting prognosis. My Father had to get my attention and let me know He was still in charge and He knows what is best. God took away my coloring book and colors until I relented and realized what He said had to be done. I had to turn the future over to Him, wait, and see what He has planned. I truly believe He

*listened to my cries and I believe He has given me an
assurance that He knows what is best and He will work all
things out as He sees fit.*

*I believe God has given my coloring book and colors
back. I have seen Ryan smile and laugh, I have seen him
cry and throw a fit. I have seen Ryan be a little boy once
again, something I did not know if I would ever see again
when I left here 10 days ago. As God has taken my hand
and guided me as I have colored the past two days, He has
shown me a beautiful picture: the picture of a little boy
who has desires and determination and parents who love
him unconditionally, standing by his bedside and doing
whatever they can to help him get by each day. Ryan gets
stronger each day, and Chris and Andrea get stronger as
well. Trying to stay strong and make sure Ryan does for
himself what he should and helping him with those things
he cannot do right now. Life has been chaotic these past
few weeks, but support has been overwhelming. However,
life continues.*

*I believe this Thanksgiving Day has been the most
special in my entire life. I have a greater understanding of
what being thankful is about. Of all of the places in this
whole world I could have been today, I don't know that
there would have been anywhere quite as special as a small
hospital room overflowing with family surrounding a truly
incredible little boy. To paraphrase an old hymn, "we don't
know about tomorrow, but we know who holds our hand."*

*I guess this has been a long read, but it flows so freely
from a grateful heart. I hope you have all had a great
Thanksgiving. This one was not what we would have
planned I am sure, but it is truly a blessing to know we
haven't celebrated it alone.*

*Now where did I put my coloring book and colors? I
have some beautiful pictures to have God help me with.*

I knew that entry was going to make people cry, but I desperately
wanted to be faithful to God, to present what I believed He wanted me
to share. As I read and re-read that entry over the ensuing months, I
gained such peace about Ryan's life. I know the entry touched other
lives as well. I was exhausted after a day in the hospital and the
emotional drain writing that entry brought with it. I had talked Nonna

into getting up and going Christmas shopping at 5:00 a.m. the next morning, so I headed for bed. For a few hours at least, I slept very peacefully.

Nonna and I had a tradition of going shopping for the "Black Friday" early morning sales. Since Ryan was better, we decided it would be fun to continue the tradition. All throughout Thanksgiving Day, we had looked through the advertisements and had made shopping lists. We laid out a plan of which stores opened earliest and where we needed to be at which time. Laura went with us and drove. We had planned to shop until mid-morning and then, Laura and I, along with our kids, were going to go to her mother and father's house in Missouri to spend some time. Since we were going to shop for a while then head out, we told Ryan goodbye on Thanksgiving Day. We told him we would not see him on Friday. He was okay with that.

Our shopping trip went very well, and we purchased many bargain priced Christmas gifts that day. Right on schedule, we finished shopping and headed out of Little Rock. It took us about three and a half hours to get to my in-laws' home.

After we arrived at our destination, I got a phone call from Chris. "After you all left town, Ryan had physical therapy."

I thought to myself, "And that is big news because…", but I didn't say anything.

Chris continued, "While he was being wheeled to therapy, he saw a tricycle. Ryan wanted to know if he could ride it. The therapists told Ryan that if he would do all of his therapy, they would sit him on it and see how it went from there."

"Well, he should enjoy riding that some day," I interrupted.

Gleefully, Chris interjected, "He did. The therapists wanted to get a baseline of what Ryan could do, so they worked him hard. Ryan did everything he was asked to do, and then he asked again if he could ride the trike. One therapist said, 'If you can walk over to it, I will put you on it.' Ryan held the hand of the therapist and slowly walked the entire width of the room, the first steps he had taken since his surgery, to where the trike was. True to his word, the therapist sat Ryan on the trike and then wrapped some gauze around his left foot so it would stay on the pedal. Ryan started pedaling, and the trike started going. He used his right leg mostly. He pushed the pedal down and when it rolled back to the top, he would push it again. It worked his left leg though, because it was tied to the pedal so it went up and down and all around."

Chris had a little more to say, mostly small talk. He was very excited, and with good reason. We talked for a few minutes, and then he had to call someone else. I hung up the phone and pondered what had happened over the past few days.

Ryan continued to impress the doctors and therapists with his drive and determination. We had continued to pray Ryan would be able to gain as much strength and mobility as possible. It would have been very easy for God to touch Ryan and restore his body completely. However, that hadn't happened. Instead, God gave Ryan an incredible desire to get better. Ryan wanted to get getter and he was not afraid of the hard work it required. As Ryan worked harder to get better, more and more people were touched by his tenacity. It gave us the opportunity to praise God for how He continued working in Ryan's life. If God had instantaneously healed Ryan, it would have been great, but it would not have touched people in the same way. Ryan became an inspiration for all of the therapists and doctors and nurses. He became an inspiration to those who were reading the website. He was an inspiration to numbers of people. God worked IN Ryan's life, but just as importantly, He worked THROUGH Ryan's life.

Ryan never once complained about the amount of therapy, the walk across the room or having to be tied to the tricycle. Ryan was thrilled to be able to ride that tricycle and when he did, he amazed everyone. I would have loved to have been in Little Rock to witness this event, but I could not be at the hospital all of the time. It just seemed a little ironic that the first time I left Little Rock, Ryan awakened from his chemical coma. This time when I left Little Rock, he had walked across the room and ridden a tricycle down the hall. He seemed to be saving his best "tricks" to perform after I was gone.

Ryan had a very long day, but the progress had been utterly astonishing. He was laughing and playing with people; he had ridden the tricycle and completed all of his therapy. He was spending time with his sissy as well as his family and friends. The only sour note of the day was the loss by the Arkansas Razorbacks football team.

On Saturday after Thanksgiving, we made the trip back to our home. When we arrived at home, I read the website to see what Chris had shared. I found that Ryan had made the trek to the computer lab along with his dad and had sent a message to all of the readers. Ryan thanked everyone for their love and prayers in a truly emotional entry. In addition, he wanted to let everyone know that he had ridden the tricycle that day as well. He had determined in his heart that he would do whatever therapy was required of him so he could do the thing he wanted to do the most: ride the tricycle. He did not realize when he was riding the trike, he was doing even more therapy. Nobody told him the difference because the harder he worked, the better he would get. Riding the trike became an ongoing part of his therapy, one he truly enjoyed.

It was hard to believe another Saturday had arrived. This Saturday marked three weeks since Ryan's surgery and two weeks since he had awakened from his chemical coma. After spending a full week unconscious, Ryan had awakened and taken the world by storm. Doctors and nurses were impressed by how well he was doing. Chris took Ryan around the hospital to visit all of the people he had become acquainted with during his stay. The nurses in the PICU were literally stunned at how much Ryan had progressed. They had seen him at his very worst. There were days when they must have breathed a sigh of relief that he had survived through their shift.

I would think one of the hardest parts of these very special people's jobs would be when a child did not survive. Some of the comments that were made while I was in Little Rock led me to believe they would not have been overly surprised if Ryan had not survived. These people worked with the most critical of all patients in the PICU. I had been told they had seen things that could only be explained by a miracle. Ryan was most definitely one of those miracles.

The week following Thanksgiving would be a week of transition. Beginning on Monday after Thanksgiving Day the therapy schedule began in earnest. In addition to the therapy, Ryan began to attend the school they had in the hospital. Outside of the therapy sessions, Chris worked with Ryan on a continual basis. If Ryan wanted something, Chris would bargain with him. Chris would have Ryan lift his left hand or arm five times or possibly more if Ryan wanted something. Ryan always got whatever he worked to obtain. Chris got the satisfaction of knowing Ryan was getting stronger. Chris was trying to get Ryan to exercise the muscles, especially on his left side. Chris would help Ryan stand and then he began working on helping Ryan walk. Within a few days following the Thanksgiving weekend, Ryan began walking as much as possible, with someone helping hold him steady.

I had tried to express some concerns to Chris while I had been in Little Rock over the holiday weekend. I was concerned he would cater too much to Ryan, giving him the impression he did not have to try. When I witnessed the way Chris worked with Ryan, I knew Ryan was going to have to work at it to keep moving forward. Ryan would not be given a free ride. He would have to work, and work hard, but in the long run he was the benefactor all the way around.

As Ryan began getting strong enough to walk with assistance, the therapists decided it would be best to make a brace to put on Ryan's leg. The concern was if they did not have him in a brace, he would turn his ankle. They were concerned if he turned his ankle it could cause him to fall and possibly hit his head. He could also damage his ankle turning it, so to avoid this whole dilemma, the brace was ordered. It had to be custom fit to Ryan's leg, so it took a few days to get it made.

On Tuesday morning following Thanksgiving, the doctors' panel met. During the meeting, the discussion of Ryan was quite exciting apparently. Though the doctors were all amazed at Ryan's progress, they were more impressed by his "bring it on" attitude. The therapists reported when they deemed Ryan to have had enough, he would not stop. He worked harder and longer than the therapists requested and he did it all with a smile on his face. They were extremely pleased with his progress. Ryan's appetite was strong and this was a good sign. The doctors warned Chris and Andrea that the upcoming chemotherapy and radiation would sap his strength and he needed to build up his body mass as much as possible before the treatments began. The steroids he was taking helped with the appetite, but I really imagine genetics helped more than the steroids.

Six is a difficult age for many kids. They want to play and they want their way; they are learning at rapid rates and they become more aware of the world around them. There seems to be an increase in the level of independence that a six year old begins to show. At the beginning of the kindergarten year, most kids start school very immature and by the end of the year they typically have learned a lot about discipline, order, appropriate behavior and a whole myriad of other lessons. While Ryan was in the hospital, he did not have an opportunity to learn many of those lessons like the other kids. However, Ryan had already matured much more rapidly than any kid should. The fact that Ryan had the attitude he did was in itself an amazing feature. Ryan did not want to back down from any challenge the therapists had to offer. Most of the time, he would meet their challenge and then move beyond the challenge just to prove he could do it. His "bring it on" statement became a slogan our entire family adopted.

The only thing Ryan really complained about in his treatment was getting "sticked." Getting "sticked" involved the drawing of blood and the giving of shots. Nearly every day Ryan was stuck by a needle, and some days, multiple times. He hated the needle pricks and since he was finally stable, the doctors decided to put a portacath in Ryan's body. A portacath was a device implanted under the skin, which used a catheter to connect the port to a vein. The port had a septum in it, which stopped all fluid from flowing outward. When a needle was inserted through the septum, medicine could be injected directly into Ryan's blood stream. If blood was needed for a test, a needle could be inserted into the septum and when a syringe applied a vacuum, the blood would travel through the needle into the collection container. If the port was not used for a time, the skin would grow over the end of the port and it was not apparent that it even existed. In Ryan's case, he had a long way to go before the portacath could be de-accessed so the skin could grow over it. For the time being, a needle would be inserted into the septum and an IV line attached to the needle. A shutoff valve would be added to the IV line to prohibit the blood from flowing backwards. The line would be taped down to Ryan's chest and every time blood work would be done, a needle would be inserted into the line, the shutoff valve opened and blood drawn without a new needle stick. Medicine would be done the same way, except a syringe would push the medicine into the body. Again, no new needle sticks. Ryan was more excited about the portacath addition than any other medical step along the whole path. Once the portacath was in place, Ryan would not really complain about anything else during the remainder of his recovery.

Ryan told the doctors the "Bad Bugs" were gone from his head when they asked how he felt. For the first time in his life, Ryan was actually able to relate what was going on inside of his head. Ryan's tumor had been growing for some time and he never really had a chance to understand what a normal headache felt like. Ryan had complained about headaches throughout his life, but he never could really explain it was more than just a headache. He was experiencing some neurological things we cannot even really begin to understand. Following the surgery and the relief from the pain he had been with for so long, he was able to try to express what it had felt like. The description was childlike, but then again, Ryan was six and it was a fitting description for what he was trying to describe.

Ryan's brace was completed, and with his brace in place, Ryan felt ready to go. Chris was pretty nervous about Ryan's stability still, but the fact that Ryan was on his feet was so much of an improvement that Chris would have gladly taken a minor fall anytime over Ryan's condition just a few weeks before. In less than one week, Ryan had gone from the wheelchair bound little boy I had seen at Thanksgiving to a little boy with a brace who was up and walking around. The brace was a huge blessing, because it gave Ryan the stability he needed, but allowed him to have more of his independence, which he also needed.

The day after Ryan received his brace, he received his port. With the port came a huge amount of freedom. Ryan would not be tied down with IVs, he was able to walk with his brace, and he was getting stronger with each passing day. When Ryan went to surgery to have his port inserted, the doctors let him push the button that added the anesthesia to his IV line. During the transport to the operating room, Ryan laughed and entertained the nurses the entire trip. I wondered how any little boy who was going to surgery could laugh about anything? It was this type of courage Ryan was exhibiting as he went under the anesthesia that made him a favorite of all the staff with which he came into contact.

The doctors, nurses and therapists all viewed Ryan with amazement. We heard on more than one occasion that they had never seen any child with the attitude Ryan exhibited. Personally, I believe Ryan's attitude was a huge factor in the progress he was making. At any point, he could have lain down, said it was too much, and given up. Instead of giving up, he seemed to thrive on the challenge. When we told anyone about his progress and how well he was doing in his recovery, they would simply shake their heads in disbelief. No one, not a single person I ever spoke with or heard from, could believe how courageous this little guy was. In a hospital like ACH, there are brave little fighters at any given time. Ryan seemed to be leading a charge against sickness. As other parents heard about his progress, they rejoiced with Chris and Andrea. Ryan's family stood in awe at the miracles God continued to perform in Ryan's life with each passing day. I truly came to believe the adage, God plus one equals a majority. That held true with each day. No matter how bad the beginnings of this journey were, each day had become a joy to witness the progress that Ryan was making.

Food had suddenly become a central part of Ryan's life. He had been a typical six-year old. He had his favorite foods, did not eat a lot at any one time, and would not try some foods just because of what they looked like. With the addition of steroids to his medicines, his appetite had become voracious. He suddenly began eating from the time he got up until he went to sleep at night. He would plan what he wanted to eat for the next day. As he was going under the anesthesia, he had already begun to make plans for what he would have when the NPO order was removed following his procedure. Ryan did not like being NPO, and I could understand why. NPO was shorthand for "Nil per os", a Latin term which roughly translated "nothing by mouth". Not only could Ryan not have food, he couldn't have anything to drink when he was NPO. Every time Ryan was to be sedated, they required that he be NPO starting at midnight the previous night. When they sedated him early in the morning, it was not too bad. However, when they kept him NPO until the afternoon, Ryan had a tendency to get a little testy.

I spoke with Chris midway through the day and Ryan had made it through the port insertion with no problems encountered. Before I called Chris, he had found out that the chemotherapy and radiation treatments were on the very near horizon. He was still unclear of what the process was going to be, but he told me that they were going to get Ryan mapped out for radiation the next day. I asked him what that meant and he really did not understand how to explain it. Basically, he understood that the mapping process told the doctors where to aim the radiation ray. I wanted to understand what he was talking about better, but he did not really have any information he could share with me at that time.

Ryan had his port inserted during the morning, returned to his room to eat lunch, and went to therapy that afternoon. During his therapy session that afternoon, Ryan decided he needed to start walking with a walker instead of having to hold someone's hand. The therapist checked him out to make sure he could walk with a walker and when he did it successfully, Ryan was able to walk back to his room under his own power, using the walker to steady himself. Yet another big day had passed. Ryan had his port, he had gotten to eat pizza, and lastly he had started walking with a walker.

The port insertion and walker addition happened on the last day of November in 2006. It was rather appropriate that as the month of November was ending and a new month was beginning we would see a change in the story of Ryan's life. The month of November had been battle for survival. Ryan had lived through one critical portion of his young life. Our hope was that Ryan had moved beyond survival.

As December dawned, we knew Ryan was going to begin his chemotherapy and radiation within a few days. We knew treatment for the cancer that remained in Ryan's head would begin to take center stage. He had made significant gains in his physical and occupational therapy by the end of November. It was unfathomable to believe that when the month of November had begun, Ryan was a little boy with a sinus infection, so we thought, and by the end of the month, he had literally become a medical marvel.

Every one of us had heard horror stories about how patients handled chemotherapy or radiation therapy. Ryan was to undergo them simultaneously. We assumed that there would be numerous problems and side effects during the treatment. None of us wanted to witness Ryan undergo the treatment for cancer, but we knew that without treatment, he would not remain with us for long. Once again, we sent out the call for prayer support and people around the globe were faithful to that call. Notifications were posted in the CaringBridge guestbook, assuring us that people were praying for Ryan's cancer therapy. And so, we were set to begin the next phase.

The light which came with the morning of December 1, allowed us to see a new curve in the path on which Ryan was traveling. As with most curves, we could not see what the path was like on the other side. However, we knew without continuing to travel the path, Ryan's journey would soon end. With considerable apprehension, we rallied behind Ryan and, as a group, we tentatively began to walk along the path, entering the bend that lay before us.

Chemotherapy and More

We found out Ryan was to have his head "mapped" on December 1, 2006. Beyond that, we did not have a clear picture of what would happen. Part of the reason for the confusion about the radiation treatments was the radiation treatments would not take place at ACH. The treatments would actually take place at CARTI. For a long time, I did not know what CARTI meant, but I found out it was an acronym for Central Arkansas Radiation Therapy Institute. The hospitals in the area all worked together and when a patient needed radiation, they went to CARTI. This meant there was not a need for each hospital to have its own radiation center. On that first day, Ryan made the first of many trips to CARTI to begin the process of radiation treatments. He had his radiation mask formed and he was "mapped" for treatments.

The procedure for making the mask was fairly straightforward. A plastic material was heated to make it pliable. Ryan had to lay still and strips of this warm material were laid across his face, making a lattice mask. The technician told Ryan it would feel like warm spaghetti. Once the strips were in place, they were allowed to cool. When the mask cooled, it turned hard. Two holes were then drilled into flange pieces at the sides of the mask, one on each side of Ryan's head. Bolts were then placed through the holes and the mask was bolted to the radiation table. Since the mask was custom fitted to Ryan's face, it held his head perfectly still. The computer, which controlled the actual radiation, was then programmed to shoot the beam of radiation into Ryan's skull, targeting the precise location of the remaining tumor in Ryan's head.

Ryan was NPO prior to having the mask made. The concern was if Ryan had not been able to lie still while the mask was created, he would have to be sedated. The NPO order was a precaution, in case they had to sedate Ryan to complete the mask. Like most things Ryan attempted, he did very well. Ryan played opossum and lay completely still while the mask was made. The time involved in making the mask was much longer than the actual radiation treatments would be. After Ryan did so well having the mask created, the doctor said he believed Ryan would be able to undergo the radiation treatments without having to be sedated. No sedation meant no NPO order on the days Ryan had radiation treatments. He could eat breakfast each morning before he went to CARTI. Everyone was thankful for that piece of information, especially Ryan. When Chris took Ryan to CARTI, for the mapping session, he found out Ryan was scheduled to have the radiation treatment just before 11:00 each morning. If Ryan had been NPO every day until almost noon, it would have been much more difficult to get him to cooperate. As it turned out, he was such a great patient this did not become an issue.

The first Saturday of December, Jenti and Shannon took more of Ryan's cousins to visit him. They had not been able to make the trip at Thanksgiving and so they had not seen Ryan since before the surgery had taken place. On that Saturday, the kids all gathered and were able to play together for the entire weekend. By this time, Ryan was able to walk to the playroom instead of having to be in a wheelchair. A very short amount of time had passed since Thanksgiving, yet Ryan had made huge strides in getting around.

While the kids played, the adults were able to sit around and marvel at how far Ryan had come since the first part of November. Shannon had not seen Ryan since the weekend of his operation. She had seen him the night of the surgery, but she had left the next day, before the battle to regulate his pressures had begun in earnest. Though she had missed all of the daily drama that first week, she had seen Ryan on one of his worst days. She was extremely moved to see him up and about. I understood completely. If one had not witnessed how horrible Ryan looked lying in the bed with all of the monitors and IVs and tubes, which sustained his life, they could not understand the true nature of the miracle of seeing him up and walking around in less than one month. I had gotten to witness this miracle at Thanksgiving, but Ryan was not walking then. I could imagine the looks on the kids' faces when they first saw Ryan. I had seen my own kids' faces when they first saw him post-surgery. I knew the feelings of amazement at seeing him up and around, I had experienced them myself. I was not physically in Little Rock, but I had been there recently enough to understand what was happening and I was so thankful God had brought Ryan to this condition. I was amazed at how determined Ryan was to get better. God was faithfully building strength in this courageous little boy, but this little boy had determined he would get better and have his life back again. Jenti, Shannon and the kids, Li'l Steve, Devonta, and Brittany, stayed through Sunday lunch and then they went home.

As a new week was beginning, everyone began to hold their collective breath again. We all wondered how Ryan would handle the chemotherapy and radiation. The doctors warned Chris and Andrea the chemotherapy drug was something they could not use for more than two years. If it was used for longer than that, it could stop helping and possibly start causing other problems. Another warning the doctors gave Chris and Andrea was the radiation could cause a loss of hearing or vision, because of the location they had to radiate. Yet another warning was the radiation could potentially cause other types of cancer to develop. Long story short, there was no way to predict how Ryan would react. Anyone who has had a loved one, or a co-worker, or possibly they themselves, who has experienced chemotherapy and radiation, knows the side effects of these treatments are often debilitating. Nausea, vomiting, weakness, weight loss, loss of hair, and the list of possible side effects went on. While we were all anxious to get Ryan started on the treatments, none of us wanted him to undergo the side effects. We were praying and we called upon God's children around the world to pray for Ryan as he was approaching treatment.

The nutritionist informed Chris and Andrea on what types of food they should try to get Ryan to eat. Protein and carbohydrates were the target items. The carbohydrates would give him energy but the protein would help him stay stronger. They did not want him loading up on a bunch of sugar and fluff junk foods. They wanted him eating substantial foods to help his body stay as strong as possible. At this time, he was not having any problem with that. He would eat, then eat again and then have a snack. The doctors were impressed with his appetite, but then they would look at his dad and realize this was only a natural progression. One thing about our family, we have always loved food, and Ryan was getting into the swing of eating. It was helping him to build strength and so all was going well. Ryan was weighed on Monday before his treatments began and he weighed all of forty-seven pounds.

Just prior to starting chemotherapy and radiation, Ryan began to wear regular clothes again. Since Ryan had gone into the hospital, he had been in hospital pajamas, if he was able to wear clothes at all. When he was back in the PICU those first weeks, he did not have any clothes on while they had him on the chilling blanket. He would be covered very minimally, to give him a little privacy, and there were no pajamas on his little body. As he had progressed, he had moved up to wearing hospital pajamas. Hospital pajamas are different from any other pajamas because they are made in a fashion that enables them to be unsnapped in any number of ways so that doctors and nurses can access their IVs, wounds, or whatever portion of patients' bodies that needed attention. Ryan was now moving beyond the point of needing the hospital pajamas, as he was finally past the IVs and he was able to go to the bathroom instead of using a bedpan or urinal. As he was able to get up and around, he was able to wear his own clothes again. It seems like a small thing to most people, but to the psyche of a six year old, it was a huge thing. Heartbreakingly, Ryan announced one day after he was allowed to wear a T-shirt and sweatpants, that he was now a "normal" boy again because he could were real clothes.

On Wednesday, December 6, 2006, Ryan went once again to CARTI and had his first radiation treatment. The target completion date for all treatments was January 18, 2007. The plan was to radiate Ryan mid-morning and give him his chemotherapy at night before he went to bed. Ryan went to the radiation room, lay on the bed where they bolted his faceplate to the table, and then as he listened to one of his favorite CDs, they administered the radiation. He never flinched and the treatment went without any glitches.

Following the treatment, Chris quizzed Ryan, "So Ryan, how did the treatment go?"

Ryan looked at his dad and said, with a smile, "It was easy peasy, lemon squeezy. Really it wasn't any different than getting an X-ray."

Though Ryan had taken a huge step forward in his treatments by getting that first radiation treatment, he did not get off easy. Therapy was an important part of each day, both physical therapy (PT) and occupational therapy (OT). The two types of therapy were so entwined most people commonly referred them as PT/OT. In addition to those types of therapies, Ryan had to undergo speech therapy, once a week. Speech therapy helped to strengthen the throat muscles, which enabled him to speak. Therapy sessions did not stop just because Ryan had started his radiation therapy. It would not be put on hold the next day either, when he began chemotherapy. PT/OT was essential in helping re-establish his muscle control. He did not complain though, he kept going and going and going. Even Ryan had a fatigue point though. He missed one of his afternoon therapy sessions on the day he began radiation. That was an exception though, not the rule.

I spoke with Chris shortly after they returned from CARTI to ACH. While we talked, I asked him about the chemotherapy treatment that was to begin the next day.

"It is some wicked stuff," he began. "The person preparing the medicine has to wear a mask, gloves, safety glasses, and protective gown. They have to go into an isolated area where they break open the capsules and dissolve the contents in apple juice. Ryan has to drink this mess, and then more juice is added to the solution, to make sure he gets all of the medicine. The empty capsules have to then be placed in a biohazard bag and sealed up. The biohazard bags then have to be incinerated."

The instructions for preparing the chemotherapy were thoroughly explained, because at some point in the future, Ryan would be discharged from the hospital. If he were still taking the chemotherapy, Chris or Andrea would have to mix the medicine for him to take. It sounded ominous, but the first time I saw it done, it looked even scarier than it sounded.

One of the hardest days for Chris happened the day after Ryan started chemotherapy. As Ryan had done so exceptionally well, Chris had decided to go back to Pea Ridge and stay with Ashtyn. Life in Pea Ridge had not stopped because of what was happening in Little Rock. People had been filling in and helping handle things in Pea Ridge while Chris and Andrea were in Little Rock. It was time for Chris to go back home and begin managing his household. In addition, he decided to return to work so if he needed more time off later into Ryan's recovery, he would still have some time available.

As he went to bed his last night at the hospital, he had the bittersweet knowledge that the next day he would be going to his own home. The next night he would be sleeping in his own bed. It was bittersweet because he was torn between wanting to get his life back to normal and leaving his son behind. It was not an easy decision, but with the excellent progress Ryan had recently made, it seemed the most prudent decision to be made. Since Ryan had breezed through the first chemo and radiation treatments, Chris decided it was time to leave Little Rock and go home.

Along the way from the initial night in the hospital in Little Rock, people had come and gone. It was time for Chris to leave and go home. There were three of the Mondy clan remaining in Little Rock: Ryan, Nonna, and Andrea. I called to see how things were going in Little Rock after Chris' departure. I was pleasantly surprised when Ryan answered Andrea's phone.

"Well hello, Mr. Ryan," I began.

"Hi, Uncle Tim," Ryan chirped.

"So what have you been up to today?" I queried.

"I got to eat breakfast with Santa Claus this morning."

"Really, did you ask him for lots of toys?" I continued.

"Some."

"So what else is going on? I hear you are taking your new chemotherapy medicine. How is that going?"

"It's pretty bad," he began. "But if you drink it all right down and then take a quick drink of Sprite or Coke, it doesn't taste too bad. They give it to me in a shot, so it goes in pretty quick."

"A shot?" I was confused. I thought it was supposed to be oral.

"Yeah, they put it in the tube and shoot it into my mouth," he replied.

Then I understood. They were mixing the medicine with the juice, putting that mixture in a plastic syringe, without a needle, and then using the syringe plunger to push the liquid into Ryan's mouth. I had seen liquid medicine given to kids that way before, when I thought about it.

Typically, I am not very good at carrying on a conversation with children, but it was just so easy to talk with Ryan. There was so much that intrigued me about how he was handling everything. I was very interested in his reactions to the whole situation. I was amazed at his maturity about everything. His explanation about how they administered the chemo drug was very helpful.

On December 9, 2006, Ryan was able to do something he had not been able to do since his surgery. He was able to take a bath. A bath to most children is not a miracle, or even a desire, but to Ryan it was a great joy. For the first time in over one month, he was able to get into a tub of water. He had to keep his portacath lead dry, so he couldn't take a shower. He didn't complain about wanting a shower, he focused on enjoying the bath.

After having his bath, Ryan was sitting in bed and Nonna was eating her dinner.

Ryan looked over at her, "What are you eating, Nonna?"

"Chicken fried steak."

"Can I have a bite?" he wondered.

"Sure thing sweetie," Nonna answered as she rose to put some on a plate for Ryan.

He took a big bite and his response was rather humorous. "Nonna, I am not sure what you are eating, but it is not fried chicken."

Nonna burst into laughter, and then she apologized for laughing. "No honey, it is not fried chicken, it is a fried steak."

"Well, I prefer fried chicken," he announced as he continued stuffing the chicken fried steak into his mouth. Then they both began to laugh and to enjoy the moment.

Ryan started having fun with his nurses about that time also. Someone gave Ryan a bag of Hershey kisses and when one of the nurses would enter the room, he would yell "Heads Up" and then start throwing kisses at them. They had great fun with that. I spoke with Ryan on the phone while he was doing this and as he was telling me about what he was doing, he hung up on me. Uncle Steve, Jenti's husband, had taught him this trick and he thought it was great fun. He would be talking and say something like "and you know what else" then disconnect the phone. It was apparent his sense of humor was shining through and everyone was enjoying seeing and hearing him being mischievous and playing tricks on people.

It seemed as if there was not a day that passed without Ryan making some huge stride in recovery. Every day he would add extra to his therapy session, or excel in some other fashion. The next huge adjustment began for Ryan when he decided he did not need a walker to help him any longer. One afternoon after he returned to his room from therapy, he was sitting on one of the chairs in his room. Nonna was sitting in another chair and Ryan decided he wanted to sit with her. He stood up, walked across the room, and sat down beside her. Then he looked at her out of the corner of his eye to see if she was going to say anything about what he had just done. Nonna just smiled, and hugged him and from that point forward, he did not use a walker anymore. He was once again free to roam about at his own pace, without any aid in walking, except for the brace to support his ankle.

He did begin to get a bit over active though. Following his occupational therapy and physical therapy sessions one afternoon, Nonna helped him get into his bed and as she stepped away to wash her hands, Ryan began to move around, trying to re-orient himself in the bed. Nonna had apparently left the bed rail down and Ryan fell out of bed, hitting his head as he fell. Panic set in. Fortunately, this occurred only minutes after one of the doctors had walked out of the room. Nonna stepped to the door and got the attention of the nurse who got the doctor. Ryan got a small cut on his ear, but no further damage. It did underscore that there were limits to what he was able to do on his own. He had made great strides, but he still did not have the muscle control he had once possessed. The little episode seemed pretty traumatic, but in retrospect, it could have been just the signal Ryan needed. He had to learn how to maintain a balance in pushing his therapy and being cautious about his body.

As Ryan was staying on the rehabilitation floor, he did not have direct access to the deliverance of his chemotherapy medication. He was supposed to get the medicine at night, but as it had to be prepared on one floor and then delivered to him on another floor. The medicine was not delivered very early in the evening and as such, Ryan had to stay up later than normal to get his medicine. The later nights mixed with early morning blood work was causing the poor little guy to be overly tired during some days. On those days, he would have to back down on his therapy, something he did not like doing. Everything was a series of adjustments. If Ryan was too tired for therapy, he needed rest. If he was hungry, he needed food. If he felt like doing therapy, he would push as hard as possible for as long as possible. There was no set pattern, only general guidelines.

The morning of December 12, 2006, the doctor's panel met. It was a momentous meeting, because during the meeting they determined it was time for Ryan to be discharged from the hospital. He would leave the hospital on Saturday, December 16, and he would reside in the RMH, with Nonna and Andrea, for the remainder of his chemotherapy and radiation. It had been nearly six weeks since the whole ordeal had started. In those early days, there were many times we did not know if Ryan would ever get out of the hospital alive. Ryan had come so far in such a short time. He had progressed in his therapy to the point he was much stronger than when we had seen him at Thanksgiving. His mobility was a factor in his ability to leave the hospital and go to the RMH. We all knew Ryan was truly getting better with each day because if he hadn't been progressing, the doctors would not have wanted to let him out of the hospital. The McDonald house was actually just about a block from the part of the hospital in which Ryan was staying, but that one block might as well have been ten miles. Being out of the hospital was a goal that had been discussed for a while and it was finally on the radar screen for the doctors, as well as the family.

In the final preparation for Ryan leaving the hospital, various tests were performed to give a benchmark for measuring future progress. He had an auditory test, which indicated his hearing was at one-hundred percent. His hearing had not been diminished from his surgery or from the radiation. The same day he had the hearing test they weighed him again. He had topped fifty pounds.

Ryan had been a big fan of the movie *Cars* and people had been giving him the toy cars from the movie. The nurses kept asking him questions about what the characters' names were and where he had gotten each car. Finally, he told them if they would give him a place to have a show and tell he would be glad to give all of the information at one time. He said that everyone could come and ask any questions they had. They set Ryan up in a conference room and he was as good as his word. He explained every character and how they related to each other.

He told who had given him each car and how it had been packaged. After he finished his "prepared remarks," he opened the floor to questions from his audience. His presentation was a huge success and greatly enjoyed by everyone in attendance.

On Thursday, before Ryan left the hospital, Ryan's portacath was de-accessed. That meant they removed the external line that was attached to it. From that point forward, any time the port had to be accessed it would be by having a needle inserted through the skin into the port. The skin surrounding the port would be numbed with a local anesthetic, so Ryan wouldn't feel the insertion. The skin would heal itself, sealing the portacath shut after the needle was removed and thus there was no longer any concern about getting wet in a shower or a pool.

When Ryan found out he would be leaving the hospital to stay in the McDonald House, one of the first things he questioned was the food situation. He wanted to know what the food schedule would be and what types of food would be served. Nonna assured him she would take care of his food needs. There was a common kitchen at the McDonald House, so Nonna would cook whatever Ryan requested, within limits. Ryan loved Nonna's cooking, so that was fine with him. He just wanted to be certain there would be plenty of foods he liked to eat.

On that Friday, Ryan went around the hospital saying goodbye to his friends. He had been on several different floors and in various wards. He went to each place he had stayed and told the people that had cared for him how much he appreciated them and gave them a little Christmas gift. Chris made the trip from Pea Ridge back to Little Rock to help make the big move. He arrived on Friday night and he was astonished with the progress Ryan had made in the interim since Chris had been at home. He was most touched by the hug Ryan gave him when Chris entered the hospital. Ryan hugged him using both arms. Having that left arm wrapped around Chris' neck was a joy no one was certain would ever happen again.

Ryan walked into the Ronald McDonald House on Saturday morning under his own strength. He walked around the house and proclaimed he liked the house very much. He believed it would do just fine.

Once all of their belongings were moved from the hospital, Chris took the family all to The Olive Garden Restaurant, at Ryan's request. This was the first time Ryan had been out in public in six weeks. He was very excited about his trip out. The service was a bit slow and Ryan was so exhausted by the events of the day that he laid down in the seat and fell asleep. Chris requested they prepare the food to go and as quickly as possible. They left the restaurant and went to the McDonald House. They were concerned it might have been too much for Ryan, but after a short nap, Ryan was back up and around as he had been before the outing. He had his food warmed and he ate it, enjoying it very much.

Moving into the McDonald House meant Chris and Andrea were responsible for administering Ryan's chemotherapy medicine. That was pretty scary for them. About an hour before he could take his chemo medicine, he had to take medicine to help him stave off nausea. This meant it had to be planned out a couple of hours in advance when Ryan was going to go to bed so they could time giving him his different medications. It was a routine, which would become the norm, at least for a while.

Ryan settled into a routine very quickly. By Monday after Ryan was released from the hospital, he had a schedule in place for physical therapy, occupational therapy, radiation therapy, speech therapy, and blood work. With the Christmas holiday approaching, we had heard some people wanted to stop by the RMH to see Ryan and pass Christmas presents along to him. We had to post his schedule on the internet so people would know when it was an appropriate time to visit. He was a busy little man. Every day he had at least one form of therapy, some days three forms. He had clinic visits and he had radiation. Those were just the things that were scheduled daily. Other things continued to pop up, like the hearing test and other tests of similar nature.

Chris had gone back to Pea Ridge and he was in contact with Little Rock throughout the day and evening. Over the weekend, Chris had tried to teach Ryan how to swallow his chemotherapy medicine in the original pill form. He bought a box of "Good & Plenty" candy. The candy pieces were very similar in size to the chemotherapy pills Ryan would be taking. Chris taught him to put the candy on the back of his tongue, take a drink of water, tip his head back, and swallow. It all was a great plan, except that Ryan was not able to do it. The plan was to get him to be able to swallow the pills, and if he could learn to swallow the capsules, there would be much less preparation and special precautions to administer his medicine. Unfortunately, it did not work the way Chris had planned.

Christmas was rapidly approaching and with Ryan's release from the hospital, plans were altered as to how we would celebrate the holiday. We had all made hotel reservations, but since Ryan was not restricted to the hospital, we decided that it would be nice if we could meet in Searcy, Arkansas, at the home of Andrea's mother, Carnell Beck.

Ryan went about each day according to his schedule. He was feeling so much better, that he was getting bored with roaming around the McDonald house. There was only so much the little guy could do and he was getting tired of those things. He was also getting anxious about going to his Granny's house for Christmas.

Blood work results continued to be good and Ryan was able to keep going right though his treatments with no concerns. Well, actually, there was a concern but it was one that was so bizarre that most people couldn't imagine it. Ryan was eating so well that he continued gaining weight. A majority of people lose their appetite during chemotherapy, but Ryan's did not seem the least bit diminished because of the chemotherapy. The steroids he took to help with suppressing the swelling of the brain caused an increase of appetite. The concern was that if he continued to gain weight it might cause a problem with the mask they created for him when he started radiation. The mask was essential to hold Ryan's head exactly still in the right position to bombard the tumor with radiation. If his weight gain continued, it could cause a problem with the fit of his mask and that could cause problems in his radiation treatments.

During the week before Christmas, a series of X-rays were taken of Ryan's head. The X-rays were taken to determine if the tumor had grown beyond the radiation area. From the X-rays, which are a very inaccurate measurement compared to an MRI, it appeared the entire tumor was contained within the radiation area. This was very good news.

All was going extremely well as we entered into the weekend before Christmas. We were going to be able to celebrate together, outside of the hospital. There was not a lot more for which we could have asked. We felt so blessed to be meeting in Searcy instead of at the hospital in Little Rock.

The Home Stretch?

With the Christmas holiday came holiday travel. I preached the morning service on December 24, but the evening service was cancelled so people could spend time with their families. It was a beautiful service and an especially moving one as I was able to share about how God had blessed our family. It seemed especially appropriate to share about how God had moved so incredibly in our family. I was able to share with the congregation that this was the same God who had sent his only Son to die for the entire human race. We celebrated the birth of Jesus Christ knowing that God still cared for us and it was continually being shown to us through God's intervention in Ryan's life.

We drove to my in-laws home on Christmas Eve. We opened presents and had our big meal together that evening. Our plan was to head to Searcy early on Christmas morning to be with Ryan and the rest of our family for the day.

It was a very enjoyable evening celebrating Christmas with my in-laws, but I was getting anxious to see Ryan. It had been a month since I had seen him at Thanksgiving. When I saw him at the hospital over Thanksgiving, he was still being strapped into his wheelchair because he was not strong enough to hold himself in the chair. I could hardly contain my excitement at getting to see him out of the hospital. When I went to sleep that night, I don't think I could have been much more excited. It was still a lengthy drive to Searcy, from my in-law's house, and I knew I needed sleep; however, it was slow in coming that night. Finally, it arrived and I drifted off with much anticipation at what the next day would bring.

Early on Christmas morning my immediate family and I got up to travel to Searcy to meet with Chris and Andrea and the rest of the family at Carnell's house. Jenti had been unable to ride to Searcy with Poppa, so we went through Poplar Bluff once again to get her. We picked Jenti up and headed for Searcy. Along the way, the weather cooperated fairly well, however, there were some points where it snowed and sleeted a bit, and we wondered if we were in for serious weather conditions.

Due to space limitations at Carnell's, Chris had made reservations for us at a motel in Searcy. Our plan was to spend all day together, and then we would go back to the motel for the night. We drove straight to Carnell's when we arrived in Searcy and the celebration began. By late afternoon, everyone was tired so we took a group to the motel to get some rest. While we were at the motel, I took the opportunity to write a holiday update for the journal. It was one of the most incredible experiences I had writing in the journal. I just sat and wept as I wrote and shared the very depths of what I had shared with my family throughout the day.

MONDAY, DECEMBER 25, 2006 04:41 PM, CST

Miracle, as defined by Merriam Webster's is "an extraordinary event manifesting divine intervention in human affairs."

As we gathered around the table to eat Christmas lunch together, it was obvious that this Christmas was truly a miracle. I want to paint as clear of a picture for you as I can, so hold on.

We (Uncle Tim and family, plus Aunt Jenti), began the day very early this morning by getting in the van and driving to Searcy. We arrived just in time to walk in and smell the aroma of Christmas lunch being prepared. Green beans, mashed potatoes, sweet potatoes, ham, smoke pork, pickled okra, and the list goes on. Stepping into Granny Beck's house was like walking into any number of Christmas's of the past. Family gathered together, lunch cooking away, so many presents they were piled out into the middle of the living room. This year was different though. We had not been to Granny Beck's for Christmas before, at least I hadn't. It did not matter though. Carnell opened her home and her heart. After all, we are all family, Ryan's family.

As I looked down the table at lunch, there were many family members there, but there were some who couldn't make it. There sat Ryan, next to his dad and his Nonna, right by Granny Beck. There was a plate of food sitting before him, and a smile on his face.

"Ham or smoked pork?" Chris asked Ryan.

"Both," came his reply.

Not surprising to me, that is what I had, and they were both excellent.

"Can we open presents now?" Ryan asked immediately following lunch.

"Not until the kitchen is cleaned up," was the reply. There stood Ryan, holding a trash bag larger than he was so the Styrofoam plates could be disposed of, smiling ear to ear anxious for the presents he was about to open.

The presents were passed out, the kids took turns around the room one present at a time. Aunt Jenti brought her and Uncle Steve's present to Ryan. All eyes turned to him as he began to open the package.

A look of unadulterated joy beamed from his face as he pulled the yellow Ramone "Cars" figure from the bag. He dipped his hand back into the bag and pulled out Doc Hudson; the look came back. A third trip into the bag brought with it a guttural screech of ecstasy as he pulled out the Buzz and Woody two car set. As I looked around the room, each person was intently watching this endeavor into euphoria. Smiles and a few tears (at least in my eyes) surrounded the room. This was not because a sick little boy had a good reaction to a gift. It was because a child had received the desires of his heart and he was completely overjoyed by it. The cancer was, at least for a little bit, gone. The focus was not on chemotherapy, radiation, or therapy. The focus was on abundant joy presenting itself when Ryan opened the gift that was just what he had wanted. I am sure most of you have felt this before, the pleasure the "perfect gift" brings to both the giver and the receiver.

As the day continues, it is now time to rest and then gather again. It has been a tiring day, but it has been a beautiful day. The sky is cloudy and it has rained most of the day. The air is cold and damp. However, our hearts are warmed with the knowledge we have received a miracle for Christmas this year. Ryan can walk and talk. He is eating well and taking pleasure in knowing his family loves him. We take pleasure in watching not only him but also all of the kids open their presents. Then off they went into the other room to play while the adults opened their gifts. I personally got some nice gifts, for which I am very thankful. I don't think I will ever forget this Christmas as long as I live. It is different from any before, probably different from any to follow, but then so is each day. Tradition is wonderful, especially at the holiday season. I think we have decided on a new tradition in our family. No matter what the circumstances are, we will enjoy the time together and treasure the love we share.

I stand in awe of Ryan's progress. I was there when he came out of surgery on November 4, 2006. I was there Thanksgiving weekend and now I am here for Christmas. I have seen God work miracle after miracle in Ryan's life and in the lives of those surrounding him.

I hope and I pray you have had a blessed Christmas day today. As for us, I can't remember a Christmas quite this special. Not just because of Ryan's condition, but because I know what it is to experience pure joy. It comes from simple faith, knowing there is not one more thing I can do to help Ryan in his recovery, but that I have to trust God. I could sermonize and explain a link between Jesus birth and joy, "Joy to the World" should help you make that connection on your own. With God in our lives, we can experience true joy. I believe we are all closer to God because of the struggles we have been through this year. With a closer walk with God comes a greater level of joy.

I may never be able to repeat this time, nor would I like to repeat the circumstances that have brought us here. I treasure the day, the gifts, and the joy, which have been given this year. I thank God for allowing us to share this day with Ryan, and I pray He will allow us to continue sharing it with him for many, many years to come. I have no assurances, but, I have hope, I have peace and I have joy. My desire is that each of you reading this update can experience the same thing this holiday season.

I want to wish all of you a blessed Merry Christmas. May you find joy in knowing that God is good all of the time and that He is still on the throne in Heaven. He reigns supreme this day as every other day. I am just thankful He has allowed us this day together. Please keep us in your prayers; we cannot express how much that means to us. From the bottom of my heart, I say "Thank You" for your prayer.

Uncle Tim.

After the napping was finished, we went back to Carnell's house to gather once again for playing games and eating some more. Throughout the evening, the kids were running around playing or watching a movie. The adults sat, visited, and played games.

Around 8:00 p.m., Chris disappeared for a bit. Then he came back in from the garage. He was wearing his mask, his gloves, and his medical gown. He had been in the garage preparing Ryan's chemotherapy medicine. As wonderful as the day had been, the image of him in that garb and then watching Ryan step up and drink his medicine like the trooper he had continued to be, brought everything back to reality. It had been a wonderful day; everyone had thoroughly enjoyed the events of the day. No matter how great the day had been, the reality was Ryan was still a very sick little boy. Watching Chris walk in dressed in his protective gear made everyone cringe as we watched Ryan take his medicine. The poor little guy was drinking something that could cause cell mutations so severe his dad had to be protected. The medicine was created for that purpose. It was a gene altering medication. It targeted a particular type of cell. I don't know how it knew which cells to alter; I guess it was based in cell structure. Cancer cells are different shapes than healthy cells. I guess the medicine was created with the ability to affect only cells of certain shapes and to leave the others alone. The reality was, as evidenced by the need of protective gear, the medicine could alter cells that were considered healthy even though it wasn't supposed to work on them. That was part of the reason for the two-year limit on taking that particular medicine. The long-term effects could be detrimental rather than beneficial. The sad thing was it might not even help to alter the cancer cells in Ryan's head, but it could cause cancer in the preparer if the proper precautions were not taken.

Everyone in the room stopped for a moment to watch as Ryan drank his juice and then rinsed the medicine down with some soda. The room was quiet for the first time that day. Then as suddenly as the calm had appeared, it disappeared, as everyone went back to their visiting and gaming. The reality had returned, but as with everything else that had happened, life was going to continue.

Eventually, we all headed back to the motel. Ryan had been up and going all day long and he was completely exhausted. He was staying at Carnell's house with Chris and Andrea and since he did not want to go to bed while everyone was still there, we all thought it best to go to the motel and let him rest. We said our goodbyes that night because Chris and Andrea had to get Ryan up and head back to Little Rock on Tuesday morning so he could have his radiation treatment on schedule.

During our visit at Christmas, Ryan had a bald spot that was beginning to form. He had been taking chemotherapy and radiation for most of the month of December, so the fact that he started to loose his hair was not a surprise. Chris had shaved his own head so when Ryan's hair came out, Ryan would not be alone in being bald. At first, Ryan had thought Chris looked funny and wanted him to grow his hair back. However, as Ryan's hair continued to fall out, he decided he wanted his dad to remain bald. It had taken a few weeks into the treatment, but he finally began to show at least one typical side effect of cancer treatment.

Ryan had to return to the clinic following his Christmas break, He had to have his blood work once again, and when he went back to the hospital for his blood work, he was able to walk the block from the McDonald House to the hospital. Ryan's blood work was all very good and the doctor was curious about the special diet Ryan was eating. Ryan had continued to gain weight even though he was weeks into his treatments. He had topped out at over fifty-three pounds.

On Tuesday night, Ryan passed another milestone. On one trip to the pharmacy, Andrea had spoken with the pharmacist about Ryan. She mentioned about having to dissolve the chemotherapy medication in juice and all of the hassle involved with giving him that medication. The pharmacist told Andrea about a special cup she had for helping children take pills. Andrea had returned to the pharmacy on that Tuesday and the pharmacist had remembered to bring the cup so Andrea could have it. That night Chris worked with Ryan and taught him to use the "magic cup." With the specially designed cup, Ryan was able to swallow his chemotherapy pills one after another. From that night forward, he never had to dissolve any of his medications; he was able to swallow all of his pills and actually came to prefer taking pills to liquids for all of his medications.

Chris and Andrea spent a short week between Christmas and New Year's Day in Little Rock for treatment. They left on Friday afternoon and headed back to Searcy to spend another holiday weekend at Carnell's house with friends.

I had never even considered the last two months of the year would have occurred the way they did. As the year 2006 dawned, life was running smoothly. Our family had been together for Christmas 2005 and everyone appeared healthy. We had come through the summer and seen each other on a few different occasions. We had spent time together at Nonna's house and all was well. Then when that phone call came in November, we were all taken completely by surprise. Every parent's nightmare had happened. One of their children was critically ill. Chris and Andrea had been devastated, but I believe that with the support of our family, they had been able to stand strong. God had been so faithful through those days in November and every day after that to bring Ryan safely to the point he was at as the year ended. He was still a sick little boy, but he was up and around and getting stronger every day. His medicines appeared to be working and he was doing well with his therapy. Each day that passed brought with it a new challenge. With each new challenge being conquered, strength was gained.

We had all been raised going to church and learning that Jesus loved us. During those last two months of 2006, we had learned, with incredible clarity, just what the Bible meant when it said He would never leave us, nor forsake us. Even in the darkest of hours we felt the strength of God's people praying. The congregation I pastored was incredible to support my wife and me, and they prayed fervently for Ryan on a daily, even an hourly basis. Outside of our church, other churches around the world were praying for Ryan. Denominations had melted away and people of all faiths had rallied together to pray. We had witnessed miracle after miracle through those days and weeks. We tried our best to share with the world what God was accomplishing in Ryan's life, but words fell far short in describing all that had happened.

Early on, times had been very grim. There had been much pain and anguish through those weeks, and all of our family experienced it. We had cried together, prayed together, laughed together, and sat quietly together. As the year came to a close, we all prayed the next year would be a better year for us. God had been faithful though and we had made it through the most difficult of times. Though we had grateful hearts for what God had done to bring us through, none of us wanted to experience more pain and suffering. I don't think any of us were saddened to see 2006 fade away. We were anxious to see Ryan complete his radiation and get home. We were excited it was only a couple more weeks before he would leave the McDonald House. We were all very glad the worst appeared to be behind us. Most of all, we were glad to be able to look BACK on what had happened. Our hope was that the worst was behind us and the best was in front of us. It was a good thing God doesn't show us all that was headed our way. We might have given up hope prematurely. We had made it thus far in our journey with Ryan. We did not know what was to come, and that was probably a very good thing.

The New Year came and with it the hope of the future. Ryan spent the weekend at Carnell's just as planned and then returned to the RMH on Tuesday, January 2, 2007. Following Ryan's return to Little Rock, he had to go to CARTI for his next radiation treatment. However, this time there was a slight setback. It was something that had been speculated as possible; however, it was not really expected. When Ryan went for his radiation, he had gained too much weight and his mask did not fit any longer. A new mask had to be fashioned and Ryan had to go through the mapping sequence once again. The need for a new mask meant Ryan could not undergo radiation for a few days. It would cause a delay in the conclusion of radiation and extend Ryan's time to be in Little Rock by a few days.

However, the good news was outweighing the bad at that point. Though the treatment was to be extended a few days it was because of Ryan's gaining weight. He was gaining because his appetite was healthy. The doctors had warned us early on that it was not uncommon for a cancer patient to lose their appetite and lose quite a bit of weight during radiation and chemotherapy. Ryan's continued weight gain and strong blood work numbers were exciting to the staff caring for him. Multitudes of comments were made about how unusual Ryan's case was. The cancer form he was dealing with was uncommon for children to begin with, but the way his body was withstanding treatment was even more paradoxical. We continued to share with the staff about the vast number of people praying for Ryan. In many of the discussions I had with various staff, they assured me they were also praying for Ryan. One nurse went so far as to share with me, back in the PICU, she had witnessed many things in the unit that doctors could not explain. She had seen unexplainable things, but even she was shocked at the progress Ryan was making. God was working in Ryan's life in a way that defied all of the odds. For that, we were grateful, yet we did not take that for granted. Every chance we had we were faithful to share the goodness of God and how He was continuing to work miracles in Ryan's life.

The night after returning to the RMH from the holidays away, Ryan went to his dad. With tears in his eyes, he said, "Look, Dad," Ryan grabbed a handful of his hair. With a slight tug, it all came out. "My hair is coming out, can you just go ahead and shave it all off?"

I know it must have pained Chris to have to shave Ryan's head, but he dutifully complied with Ryan's request. With his own head shaved, Ryan decided that his dad didn't look so strange. Ryan came to grips with his new look rather quickly, and the fact that it was winter didn't hurt either. With the winter, he could wear a hat all of the time if he wanted.

Ryan had been an incredible patient and had made such remarkable strides in recovery that it was heartbreaking to hear him say he was concerned about how people looked at him. With the loss of his hair, the scar became very pronounced. Ryan became concerned he would scare people, especially other kids. He had been through so much, but even then, he was more concerned about scaring kids by his appearance than he was about the actual baldness.

Following the New Year's weekend, the return to the RMH brought with it a bit of a problem. Ryan began to exhibit an aggressive nature due to the steroids. He would get extremely irate, in an instant, if things did not suit him. When he got upset, he did not calm down very well. He wanted what he wanted, when he wanted it. The doctors told Andrea this was one of the side effects of the continued steroid usage. The episodes were sporadic, so it did not become a crisis. Andrea and Nonna did learn to navigate around his moods rather quickly and everyone continued to reside together in relative peace.

By Friday following New Years Day, Chris was back at work. The delay caused by the new radiation mask was only a few days and so it did not take long for Ryan's treatments to get rolling along again. Once the new mask was in place and a new target date for the completion of radiation was established, Ryan began the final countdown to going home. He was very anxious to get home and he had already started making plans to play spring T-ball with his best friend.

Ryan wanted to play T-ball. Most people who heard Ryan say he wanted to play T-ball smiled a sort of sly little smile, which seemed to say, "That's nice, but there is no way that will happen anytime soon." When Chris had returned to Pea Ridge following the New Year, Ryan coached him in how he was supposed to get Ryan signed up and placed on a T-ball team. Ryan had such a positive outlook that he never doubted he would be able to play T-ball that season. He was not dwelling on the problems of the day; he was planning. Most people dismissed this desire as a childish lack of understanding illness. However, most people forgot that he was a child who had gone from bedfast to unassisted walking in less than a month. It appeared that nothing was going to stand in Ryan's way when he decided he wanted something, and wanted to play T-ball. Chris promised to see what he could do and the topic was momentarily dropped.

Once Ryan's portacath was sealed over completely, he was able to begin his physical and occupational therapies in the pool. He really enjoyed these therapy sessions. He was also very pleased when he found out on January 5, 2007, more than 20,000 visitors had been on his website. A lot of these were repeat visitors, but the level of concern was amazing.

Weekends were now becoming more normal. If Andrea and Nonna needed to run to the store for something, they could. Ryan was able to get out and about, though not for very long periods. Over the weekend, there was no radiation or therapy, so Ryan had to find things to occupy his time. He liked to call people and talk to them, watch TV, color or put puzzles together. He helped Nonna around the kitchen on occasion.

Each Monday, Ryan would go to the clinic and have his port accessed. His blood was drawn and all necessary tests were performed. The tests were done to check how various components of his blood were responding to the chemotherapy and radiation. If the tests showed acceptable numbers, treatment proceeded as normal. If the numbers were out of line, then adjustments would be made. During those first forty-two treatments, Ryan's numbers never dropped, so we never found out what those adjustments would have been. Everything the doctors required for continued treatment was met every time. Ryan did not have to have any blood transfusions or miss any treatments because of low numbers. His numbers actually improved some of the weeks, contrary to all expectations. His weight continued to increase and his appetite did not waiver. He was by all accounts, a healthy little boy. The only problem was that pesky tumor in his head.

As the second full week of January rolled around, Ryan's weight had reached fifty-seven and one-half pounds. He had gained fifteen pounds during the weeks of chemotherapy and radiation. He started fighting a cold during the first week of January, but by the second week, his symptoms had cleared.

The hematology and oncology doctors had an MRI and a series of X-rays performed during the second week of January. The doctors told Andrea they wanted to make sure the fluid level inside of Ryan's head was what it should have been. They told Andrea these tests were merely for basic diagnostic purposes. They did not expect to find any information concerning the effectiveness of the treatments at that time. They told Andrea an MRI would be done twelve weeks after the last radiation treatment and that would be the one that gave them the information they needed. On Wednesday, January 10, 2007, we received an incredible surprise from the doctors. The MRI and X-rays done the day before were not supposed to have given a lot of information; however, they gave a wealth of information.

The radiation treatment caused swelling as one side effect. When the MRI was performed, the results showed that even with the swelling that occurred because of the radiation treatments, the tumor was smaller than it had originally been. Hematology, oncology, neurology, and radiology all conferred and it was definitive. The tumor was shrinking. Andrea also received word that it would not be twelve weeks after the last treatment; it would be two weeks after the last treatment to determine the effectiveness of the treatments.

I was ecstatic about the information. As it was Wednesday, I was able to share this information at prayer meeting that night. We sensed the presence of God that night as we poured our hearts out to Him praising Him for all He had done in Ryan's life. We had experienced yet another miracle. We had expected to wait for many weeks before we knew if the treatments had worked. God had just taken the opportunity to show us how much He was working in Ryan's life.

Then began the final full week in Little Rock. About the middle of the week, I felt led to share a picture I had taken of Ryan about forty-eight hours after his surgery. He had made such huge strides in his recovery that I wanted to show the post-op picture side-by-side with one as he was completing his treatments. I talked the situation over with Chris and Andrea and they agreed with my idea. They had never seen the picture, but they had similar ones. I posted the picture and placed a caveat on the website so people were prepared for the image before they opened the picture section of the website. The picture was truly horrific. It showed Ryan on the Monday following his surgery. All of the pumps, gauges, and monitors could be seen. The image showed him laying in the bed with the ventilator tube down his throat. Also visible in the photo was the terrible swelling that was present as a result of the surgery. We had a current picture of him and put them on the website side by side. The stark contrast was incredibly hard to believe. The three pictures that stood out on the website were Ryan's school picture, the one taken right after surgery, and the one where he had been on steroids. It did not look like the same person in any of the three pictures. He had gone from a healthy six-year-old kindergartener to the child at the doorstep of death to the rotund little figure now with us. The thing that remained the same from his school picture to the latest picture was his smile. Even though he had been through a lifetime of turmoil in the previous two months, his smile remained.

His strength throughout the chemo and radiation treatments was incredible. The doctors had not expected that. It is generally the case that, as a patient goes through chemotherapy and radiation, their blood counts drop. The patient will then have to receive blood, plasma, or platelets to strengthen his or her immune system. Ryan had made it to the end; his last clinical visit had confirmed strong numbers. He never required blood, platelets, or plasma.

Ryan's weight gain and subsequent delay in radiation treatments caused an extra weekend in the Little Rock area. On Friday, January 19, Ryan completed his radiation treatment and his family left for the weekend to go to his Granny Beck's house in Searcy. Jenti and Shannon made the trip to Searcy to meet with Nonna, Andrea, and Ryan. Chris and Ashtyn made the trip as well. They converged on Carnell's house one more time, but after that visit, Jenti and Shannon took Nonna home rather than leaving her in Arkansas.

By end of his treatments, Ryan had developed the ability to take his chemotherapy medication without the use of the "magic cup" the pharmacist had given to Andrea. He had matured to the point he could swallow all of his pills and he did not need any special tricks to do it. He just popped them into his mouth, tilted his head back, and swallowed. All he needed was a sip of water. He completed the chemotherapy ahead of the radiation, because there was no delay in chemotherapy. He finished that treatment right on the originally scheduled January 18.

Nonna, Jenti, and Shannon stayed in Searcy until that Sunday and then they went home. Chris and family stayed in Searcy that Sunday night and when they arose on Monday, they drove to Little Rock for the final radiation treatment.

Then it was over. On January 22, 2007, after eighty days away from home, Ryan completed his last radiation treatment. Chris and family all returned to Pea Ridge. He had undergone surgery, thirty radiation treatments, and forty-two chemotherapy treatments. He had gone from a week in a chemically induced coma to being able to walk about the McDonald House on his own. He ended that portion of his journey when he returned home that day in January.

Though Ryan was home, we all knew it was only a brief resting point in the journey. When Ryan left Little Rock, he already had an appointment for February 5, 2007, for the follow-up MRI. We did not know what would happen from that point, but we were overjoyed by the fact that Ryan had returned home. I called Chris the day after they returned home.

"So how did it feel to have everyone at home last night?" I asked.

With peace in his voice, Chris responded, "It was so restful. No monitors, no nurses, nothing. We were able to put Ryan to bed last night in his new *Cars* bedroom and he thought that was awesome. I don't know what the future holds for us, but I surely enjoyed last night, having everyone safely back home."

Journal entries came to a screeching halt for the most part after Ryan left the McDonald House. It just did not seem to be a priority any longer to write in the journal about what had happened each day. Life was going well. Ashtyn was in school each day and Ryan had his tutor coming to the house to help him with his schoolwork. It turned out his homebound teacher was actually his classroom teacher, Mrs. Kennemer. She would not have it any other way. When plans were being made to have a teacher come to their house, Chris and Andrea did not try to push the school for Mrs. Kennemer to be the one. However, Mrs. Kennemer insisted she be Ryan's teacher. It required extra hours and extra effort, but she took that upon herself. She wouldn't hear of anyone else teaching "her Ryan."

While Ryan was undergoing the latter stages of treatment, Chris had been in Pea Ridge with Ashtyn. Chris had returned to work during the last several weeks of Ryan's treatment, and in the evenings he had been preparing a surprise for Ryan. Chris decorated Ryan's room in a *Cars* theme. He had gone to the extent of buying a sewing machine and making *Cars* curtains for the room. When Ryan returned home, he had a very impressive room he enjoyed immensely.

I could tell that every time I spoke with Chris he was just thankful to have Ryan home. I continued to flashback to a conversation Chris and I had within the first two days after surgery. With tears in his eyes, Chris had told me he did not care if Ryan could walk or not, he just wanted to be able to take him home again. It had come true. Ryan had made it home. As an added blessing, he was able to walk. He was able to play with his friends. He was able to complain when he was not happy and he could tell them he loved them. All of those things were added blessings they did not know if they would ever get to experience when the surgery took place in November. Times were looking bright and all that remained was waiting for the next MRI to see what the doctors would tell them. They already knew the chemotherapy and radiation had been working. The CT scan and X-rays had confirmed that. They just waited for the MRI to see what was next on the journey.

I knew Chris and Andrea were going to Little Rock for the MRI on February 5, so I waited until the afternoon of that day and then I called Chris. Everything had been so incredibly upbeat during the latter stages of treatment, and I expected a very good report from the doctors. When I spoke with Chris, I found that was not the case. I did not expect the information that Chris gave me and I must admit it felt as if I had been punched in the stomach. I was crushed. We had come so far on the journey and then we had been stopped right where we stood. The report was not good and on that afternoon, we did not have a clear picture of what would transpire. What we did know was Ryan had been through more than any person, especially a child, should have to undergo. On February 5, 2007, we found that the resting point we had reached in our journey was going to afford us only a short respite. We were going to have to pick up and get going once again.

Surgery – Part Deux

The MRI from February 5 showed the tumor had in fact shrunk; however, it remained. This should not have been a shock, we knew from the previous MRI and X-rays that it was there and getting smaller. What we did not realize was that the next step in treatment was a second surgery. The doctor that Chris and Andrea spoke with on February 5 was the oncologist, not the neurosurgeon.

"Mr. and Mrs. Mondy, the tumor has started retreating due to the chemotherapy and radiation. In my opinion, our best course of action would be to perform a second surgery to remove the remaining tumor while it is retreating. The tendrils of the tumor have somewhat released their grip on the nerves that are near it. Again, in my opinion, if we do not attempt to remove the remainder of the tumor, it could do one of two things. The rest of the tumor could die as we continue the maintenance dosage of chemotherapy, or it could become aggressive once again and regain all of the ground we have recovered." The doctor paused for that bombshell to sink in and then continued, "I will have to have the neurologist review the MRI, but I believe surgery is imminent."

As Chris dispersed the word, we were all shocked. Ryan had progressed so far that it was nearly unimaginable to us that he would have to start over. In early November 2006, we had been told to expect a second surgery, but when that time had passed, we had not really considered that a viable course of treatment any longer. It was now months later and we collectively cringed at the thought of Ryan returning once again to that incredibly critical state following the first surgery.

How does one try to pray in a situation like that? If the neurologist decided not to do a second surgery that meant he did not have a hope that the second surgery would be useful. In other words, there was no hope of removing the entire tumor, so there was no need to do any surgery. On the other hand, if he determined that a second surgery was the best course of action, it meant we could very well end up back at square one. We did not know which was best, but we knew that a very critical juncture had arrived.

The evening and night of February 5, 2007, was spent in much prayer about the direction Ryan's care was to follow. We sent a request for prayer to everyone we could reach. We posted the prayer request on the website. We were at a loss as to what we wanted to happen. We determined the best thing to do was pray for God's direction for the doctors and we would all defer to their wisdom. We requested that we would have people in all fifty states once again commit to praying for Ryan. We had our "Nation of Prayer Map," however, we wanted to resurrect the assurance that the entire nation was praying for Ryan.

Midway through the afternoon on Tuesday, Chris and Andrea heard from Little Rock. The neurologist had reviewed the MRI and concurred with the oncologist. A second surgery was the best course of treatment.

The second surgery would differ from the first in a variety of ways though. The neurologist that would perform the second surgery was not the same surgeon that had performed the first surgery. The second surgery would be performed by the head of the neurology department. The piece of equipment that was not functioning in November, which had resulted in the scaled back evacuation procedure, was once again working properly. The doctor informed Chris and Andrea that when the surgeon had stopped operating in November, he had done so because he could not remove more of the tumor without causing further motor skill damage. The second surgery would attempt to remove the rest of the tumor and as such, it could cause more damage to the motor skills on Ryan's left side. Basically, Ryan had not been paralyzed by the first surgery, but he could be paralyzed because of the second surgery.

And so, on February 6, 2007, we found that Ryan would undergo a second surgery and the doctor's office was in the process of trying to work the surgery into his schedule as quickly as possible.

The prospect of a second surgery had caught us off guard, but by the time we heard back from the neurologist's office, we had our feet back under us. In November, we had been completely unprepared for what transpired. In the days following the surgery, we could tell that the prayers of God's people sustained us and brought Ryan through those horrible days. On February 7, I felt led to begin seeking prayer support in advance of the second surgery. I posted prayer requests on the website and then I sent a personal e-mail to every world area of our denomination for which I could get an e-mail address. I gave a brief account of Ryan's struggles and asked for prayer support around the world.

On February 8, Andrea received notification from the neurologist's office. Chris and Ryan were to make a preliminary trip to Little Rock on February 13, for a meeting with the neurologist and the oncologist. The surgery was scheduled for February 23. By the time Andrea spoke with the doctor's office, we had received notification that people were praying for Ryan in twenty-five states and three foreign countries.

Without any knowledge of what the future held, we did have the knowledge that people all around the country cared. Signatures in the guestbook continued to be added daily and with each added signature, our spirits were lifted. With each additional state being added, we became more confident that God was moving the hearts of His people to pray.

On Saturday before Chris met the neurologist, Ryan began suffering from an excruciating headache. Nothing seemed to help the pain. He spent the better part of the weekend in agony. As Chris made the trip to Little Rock with Ryan, Ryan lay in the seat of the van trying to rest because he felt so terrible. Chris and Andrea had taken Ryan to the hospital in Rogers, the closest hospital to their home over the weekend, but the hospital did not want to treat him due to his extensive care in Little Rock. They gave him some medicine for pain and sent him home. They recommended Chris take him to Little Rock, so that was what he had done. When Chris met with the neurologist on that Monday, the doctor explained that the steroids being withdrawn caused the headache. The oncologist had started weaning Ryan off the steroids, but it had been at a rate that was too rapid. As the steroids left Ryan's system, the brain started swelling a bit and caused a headache. The neurologist determined Ryan needed to have the steroids until after the surgery and so he gave Ryan a new prescription. Ryan was given a dose of steroids before he left the doctor's office and by the time he headed home, the headache had started to subside. Chris and Andrea were extremely relieved the headache was caused by the removal of the steroids rather than something more severe.

No significant new information was gleaned from the meeting with the doctors. We had anticipated something dramatic might be revealed during that meeting with the doctors, but really, the neurosurgeon just wanted to meet Ryan and Chris before the day of the surgery. They discussed the situation with the headache, set the schedule for the day of the surgery, and then the meeting was over. After meeting the doctor, Chris headed back to Pea Ridge and Ryan rested much more comfortably thanks to the steroids being re-introduced to his little body.

Ryan would be the first surgery of the day. He would have to be at the hospital on the morning of the surgery between 5:30 and 6:00, for the pre-op procedures. The surgery would commence as early as possible after he was prepared on the morning of February 23. One positive note from meeting the doctor was he had told Chris he believed the entire tumor could be removed with the second surgery. Our hopes were buoyed by that comment, but at the same time, we had to wonder what the cost would be in a loss of mobility.

With the steroids being back in Ryan's body, the headache began to be less detrimental. Ryan was able to get out of bed on February 14, and go to school to celebrate Valentine's Day with his classmates. I checked on him that day after school and found it had all gone very well. I also found out before he had gotten the headache the previous weekend, he had gone to work with his dad for a meeting. During the meeting, he was introduced to the approximately one-thousand employees in the audience. Later we found the meeting had been on a live feed with another fifteen-hundred people in another building witnessing the event. Ryan was introduced and handed a microphone. He looked out over the crowd and thanked them all for their kind thoughts and their prayers. According to Chris, tears flowed unashamedly across the room.

Beside Ryan, there were other guests at that meeting. One of the other guests was a former United States senator and presidential candidate. In addition to the senator, several members of the Tuskegee Airmen were present that day. After the meeting, Ryan was personally able to meet with these other distinguished guests. It had been an extremely moving day, and then the headache had struck Ryan. That passed though and Ryan was right back on track, reliving the experience and having a great time at his Valentine's party sharing his weekend adventure with his classmates.

Within forty-eight hours of beginning the steroids once again, Ryan's appetite returned and the headache completely subsided. When Ryan started feeling like getting up and around, a collective sigh of relief went through all of us. When he began to want food, we all knew he was doing much better. He was still sluggish, but at least the steroids were helping to alleviate the most severe symptoms.

With one week to go before the second surgery, I counted the number of guestbook entries with promises to pray for Ryan. On the Friday before the surgery, we had representatives in forty-five different states and twenty-eight different foreign nations. The prayer support was an incredible boost and we were getting very anxious to have the second surgery behind us at that point. I had started an e-mail campaign asking for prayer among members of the Nazarene congregations around the world. I pastored a Nazarene church in Illinois, and the Nazarene denomination has missionaries around the world. It is not safe to ask for prayer requests in certain parts of the world, where Christianity is taboo, so I contacted the educational centers around the globe and asked them to disperse the request, as they knew the safe areas to contact. It had worked, as the twenty-eight foreign nations were evidence. Ryan's case had literally become a worldwide prayer battle.

That last week before the surgery passed as a blur. On February 22, we all made the journey once again to Little Rock. I had to begin my trip earlier than everyone else did as I had farther to drive. As I drove, I could feel the presence of the Holy Spirit with me. I began to pray about the whole situation we were facing and I could tell God was giving me comfort. During that trip, I had an encounter with God, which gave me a peace about the surgery I could not have imagined.

My favorite book, other than the Bible, is a book entitled "The Lion, the Witch and the Wardrobe" (for brevity, I will call it LWW), by C. S. Lewis. You may have heard of it, as a few years ago, a major motion picture of the book was made and it drew a lot of attention to the book. Actually, there are a set of seven books and I love them all. However, this book has such rich spiritual applications that I continue to gain new insights every time I re-read it.

The weather was incredibly beautiful on the trip to Little Rock, and for a February day, it was very warm. The signs of spring were starting to appear all around. In LWW, the witch had cast a spell across the land of Narnia, which caused it to be "always winter, but it never gets to Christmas." Not to spoil the book, but at the point that the land of Narnia begins to experience a spring thaw, it happens because of the coming of Aslan (who is the personification of Jesus Christ). In LWW, finally Father Christmas comes and brings gifts to the main characters. When that happens, it is the beginning of the destruction of the evil witch. As I was traveling and seeing the signs of spring all around me, it made me ponder that portion of LWW.

It had been winter when Ryan was diagnosed. It was dark and cold when I got to Little Rock that night in November, before the coming of Christmas. As I drove to Little Rock for the second surgery, we had been through most of the winter, and spring had started to show itself. We had experienced a wonderful Christmas, and the perfect presents were a joy to share. As I was driving to Little Rock, I started to reflect on the whole episode in LWW and when the spring started to arrive, it indicated that Aslan (Jesus) was doing something spectacular. The beautiful weather of the day on which I was traveling made me realize that God had done a mighty thing already in Ryan's life and suddenly I was completely assured everything would be all right with Ryan's surgery.

The difficulty in sharing all that transpired in the van on the way to Little Rock is frustrating. It was as if I could sense the Holy Spirit laying a hand on my shoulder and telling me God was in control. I began to sing along with some praise songs that were playing on the CD player and I was so excited that I could hardly contain myself. I couldn't wait to get to Little Rock and share with everyone what I had experienced. Sadly, when I tried to re-live what I had experienced, I just couldn't put it into words.

I arrived at the motel first and when Chris got there, I was amazed to see Ryan step down out of the van all by himself. He was walking rather slowly because he did not have his brace on his ankle. He stepped gingerly down from the van and then began walking across the parking lot toward me. I have to admit, a tear escaped from my eye to witness such a blessed miracle. All of the reflections I had been having on the trip to Little Rock were immediately confirmed God was indeed in control of the entire situation.

We arrived in Little Rock at the motel within ten minutes of each other. It was amazing to see Nonna's car, Chris' van, and my van all pulling into the parking lot at almost the same time. Jenti was a little behind the rest of us, but she made it shortly after we all got to the motel.

While we waited for Jenti to get to the motel, I asked Ryan if he was nervous.

"Why should I be nervous, Uncle Tim?" Ryan wondered.

"Well, I was wondering if you were nervous about the surgery," I pressed.

At that point, he began to roll around on the bed, holding his side as he laughed extremely hard. "Why should I be nervous about that? I have already been through that and everything is fine. As long as I don't have to get sticked, there won't be any problems."

Talk about courage.

Eventually, Jenti and Shannon made it to the motel. When they got to the motel, we all went out for dinner at The Olive Garden, again at Ryan's request. It was a very nice evening. Ryan went from place to place seeing what everyone was eating, laughing, and telling funny stories. It was apparent the steroids were working, as he tasted the food of several different people as he made the rounds. He ate until he was full, then he started getting tired. We all finished eating as quickly as we could and left.

Chris and Andrea had been scheduled into a room at the Ronald McDonald House. As Ryan was an ongoing patient, they were bumped to the top of the list for a room. After we all finished eating, they took Ryan and headed for the McDonald House and the rest of us went to the motel to get some rest. I don't think anyone really rested much, but we went to bed and pretended at least.

We could not get into the hospital until after 9:00 a.m., and since Ryan had to be there much earlier, we spoke with Chris by phone after Ryan had been taken to surgery. Before 8:00 a.m., Ryan had been prepped and had already been taken to surgery. As we returned to the PICU waiting room once again on that Friday morning, we did not know how many days we would have to go through the process again. We were taking one day at a time and the first day meant we would sit in the waiting room and wait for the surgeon to tell us how the surgery had gone.

One of our newfound friends had gone the extra mile to keep up with Ryan's progress that day. She was in the Arctic Circle photographing wildlife. She had arranged with a friend in Canada to keep updated. The lady in Canada agreed to use a satellite phone to pass the updated information to the Arctic Circle. Knowing she had gone to that much trouble to keep up with Ryan's progress, we wanted to do our best to share as much information as possible, as quickly as possible throughout the day. We updated the website as frequently as we could, but there were many hours with no information. Finally, about noon we received word from the operating room that all was going as well as could be expected.

The surgery had been scheduled to last four hours. When we received the phone call at noon, it had been about four hours since Ryan had been taken to surgery. At noon, the nurse told Andrea the timetable had been lifted. Everything had been going well to that point, but the surgery was going to be a long slow process to remove the entire tumor. The surgeon would be operating until he was satisfied he had done all he could do. There was no estimate as to how long that could be. It was comforting to know the surgery was going well, but it was frustrating to know we would just have to wait and we did not know for how much longer.

With each report we received after that initial one, all continued to be going well. Ryan's vitals held strong and they had found nothing unexpected. The calls were very spread out, and we only received two additional calls throughout the afternoon. We were anxiously awaiting an update call when a doctor came to speak with the family. He had been one of the doctors who had assisted in the surgery. Rather than call us, he came to talk with us in person. He asked if the neurosurgeon had spoken with us. When we said no, he explained how the surgery had gone. We sat and listened with rapt attention. After the report, the doctor turned and walked away as if it were common to share that type of information. Within just a few minutes of the first doctor leaving, the head neurosurgeon walked in to share his insights. Mames walked in just before the main neurosurgeon started sharing with us. She got so excited when she heard his report that she started jumping up and down, up into a chair, and back to the floor a few times. She looked at us as if we were stones because we were not more excited, but then she found out we had heard the information a few minutes earlier from the other doctor.

The doctors gave us the same information, they had finished the surgery, and they had gotten all of the cancer. They were certain that all of the cancer was gone. After the doctors shared this news with us, we gathered and began to pray and thank God for what He had accomplished that day.

As we concluded praying, we looked up and there stood the head neurosurgeon. "Ryan is awake and he would like to see his mom and dad."

The surgery had utilized nearly the same incision line as the first surgery. The opening had been enlarged somewhat to reach the area that had not been operated on the first time. The surgeons had very carefully used a microscope and viewed every detail of the brain to determine which cells to remove. The surgeon removed every cell that could be seen with a microscope. The surgery had lasted about eight and one-half hours, but the surgeons were completely satisfied that the surgery was a total success.

Chris and Andrea went to check on Ryan. After a few minutes, Chris returned to the waiting room to allow others to visit Ryan. To say we were awestruck was an understatement. Following the first surgery, it had been almost a week and a half before Ryan could talk. Following the second surgery, it took just over an hour for him to be able to talk to us.

I took a turn to visit Ryan, and I was amazed. He was in such an incredibly different physical state than he had been after the first surgery that I could not believe it. As I stood and witnessed the sight, I was awash in remembering the calm assurance about the surgery I had been given on the trip to Little Rock. I carried on a conversation with Ryan that just completely astounded me. Keep in mind this dialogue occurred slightly more than an hour after an eight and one-half hour surgery.

With the surgery being on a Friday, Ryan was able to have his very favorite nurse care for him and that had excited him greatly. Ryan told Nurse Valerie he was thirsty, so she helped him get a drink of water.

"Doesn't that water taste good? It must be much better than having that tube down your throat." I commented.

He looked as though he was recalling an event from the distant past, "You know, last time they had a tube down my throat to help me breathe and a tube down my nose to help me eat."

He went on to explain the tubes should have been reversed, at least in his mind. I was impressed. He had his memory, he had the ability to question, and he was awake enough to wonder why things had occurred the way they had following the first surgery.

I went back to the waiting room and allowed others to visit Ryan. Jenti and Mames went in together to visit Ryan and they were conversing about how good he looked. He became annoyed with them and looked squarely at them and said "Girls, zip it." They quieted down and quickly left the room before they burst into laughter.

When Chris had spoken with the neurosurgeon before the operation, the doctor had not been able to give a lot of information about how much if any loss of motor skills there would be. As the evening wore on, it was apparent Ryan had not lost any of his fine motor skills. He was not only able to move his arm and his leg; he was able to move his fingers as well. Every time someone would ask him if he could move his arm or his leg, he played the helpless patient. However, when Nurse Valerie asked him something, he was like a different person. When she asked if he could move his arm or leg, it was not slight movement; he would pick it up and move it around as if there was no impairment.

Throughout the evening, Ryan's greatest disappointment was they would not allow him to have any food. He was allowed to have Sprite and water, but just before we had to leave the hospital, he vomited his water and Sprite. He was not too upset about getting sick, but he was upset because he was certain they were not going to feed him since he could not keep his liquids down.

That night when we went back to the motel, we slept a sleep that befits victors. We had been through a very long day in the waiting room, but just to be able to hear Ryan's tiny little voice following the surgery was a boost that probably would have carried us much further along the path if we had to go. Fortunately, all had gone well so we were able to go back to the motel and sleep.

When we got up on Saturday morning, we went to the hospital. The weather looked frightful, and as the morning progressed, the weather continued to worsen. The capitol building for the state of Arkansas is a few blocks from ACH, and the large windows of the PICU waiting room directly faced it. We had spent many hours staring out those windows in our two stays in the PICU. On that day, the wind and rain were so great at times that we could not see the capitol building. During the early afternoon, a tornado hit a small town south and east of Little Rock. Much of the town was destroyed and a few lives were lost, I believe. While we sat in the waiting room, we watched the storm. It was ironic though that while there was a storm raging outside, calm surrounded us within the waiting room.

Mid-morning, through the terrible wind and rain, a special visitor arrived to check on Ryan. After Chris had gotten the original pathology report, he found out about a man named Kevin. Kevin worked for the same company for which Chris worked. Kevin had suffered from the exact type and stage of cancer five years earlier. Following Ryan's initial diagnosis, Chris had made contact with Kevin. Chris had not met Kevin, but had conversed via e-mail on occasion. Kevin walked into the waiting room and introduced himself. Kevin sat and talked with us for hours. Kevin's story was not only encouraging to us, but also a phenomenal story in its own right.

Kevin had grown up about ten miles or so from where Chris, Jenti, and I had grown up. When our grandmother was alive and running her restaurant, Kevin's family would frequently come to the restaurant to eat. I had not realized it before, but Kevin's brother was the pastor of my in-laws. When Kevin had been diagnosed with cancer, his family had requested prayer, much in the same manner we had requested prayer for Ryan. We had prayed for Kevin five years earlier when he had been diagnosed with cancer. He had undergone the same surgery Ryan had undergone, he had been treated with radiation and chemotherapy just like Ryan, and had been operated on by the some of the same surgeons who had operated on Ryan. Kevin revealed to us that the head neurosurgeon who operated on him had been named the "Neurosurgeon of the Century" by the Congress of Neurological Surgeons. The assistant surgeon during Kevin's surgery was the head surgeon in Ryan's second surgery.

Kevin shared with us many, many insights we could not even imagine. He told us of the physical pain that Ryan would suffer during the coming hours and days. Kevin warned us that Ryan would be extremely sensitive to sound over the upcoming twenty-four to thirty-six hours. The worst part was when Kevin tried to describe the crackling and popping sensations that would be taking place inside of Ryan's head. As the portions of skull settled into the place where they would re-calcify, they would make all kinds of noises that could not be heard outside of the head, but he assured us they were nearly unbearable to contend with inside, where only the patient could hear them. Overall, Kevin was extremely upbeat. He praised "Dr. Jesus" for all He had done in Ryan's life.

I listened for over an hour as Kevin spoke, then as Chris and Kevin continued to talk, I went to Ryan's room. He was asleep when I got to his room, so I took a few minutes to speak with his nurse. She told me Ryan would most likely be moved out of the PICU on Sunday. They had considered moving him on Saturday; however, the inability to keep fluids down had made the doctor hesitate in moving him to a regular room. One other complication was his eyes were swollen shut. After the first surgery, the swelling had focused on the side of his head on which the incision had been made. It had taken several days to move across and down his face. Following the second surgery, the swelling had been much less severe and more evenly dispersed. The down side to that was it caused both eyes to be swollen shut at the same time.

Ryan awoke while I was talking to the nurse. I asked him how he was doing. Rather testily, he let me know he was not happy about not being able to see. "I'm blind you know," he blurted out.

"Ryan, you aren't blind," I tried to comfort him, "your eyes are just swollen shut. In a few days, after the swelling goes down, you will be alright."

"Can I see you?" He impatiently barked at me.

"Well, no you can't see me right now," I began timidly.

Rather angrily, Ryan growled, "If I can't see you, then I am blind aren't I?"

Knowing that I was losing the debate, I chatted with him for a few more minutes, trying desperately to change the subject. He was so terse I didn't want to upset him any more than necessary, so I cut the visit short and went back to the waiting room.

Other people went in to check on him and he was just as cutting with his remarks to them. Kevin overheard some of the things we were hearing from Ryan and he told us it was because of those noises inside of his head. He warned us it would probably be best if we did not visit him a lot. He recommended letting Ryan rest over everything else. So, we decided to let him rest.

It was a rather slow day since we were letting Ryan rest as much as possible. Following the first surgery, we were so concerned about whether or not he would wake up that we were constantly watching over him, praying over him, and spending time with him. This time he was so much better following the surgery that we just watched over him and prayed prayers of thanksgiving. We were all much more relaxed because he was so much better. It had not really dawned on us before, but Ryan had gone through this entire phase of recovery in his chemically induced coma. Kevin reminded us of that when we began to wonder why Ryan was so grouchy. When Ryan had awakened, he had already been through the settling of the bone fragments and the incredible pressure issues. This time, he was conscious for all of those sensations, so he had good right to be a bit grumpy.

Once the storm had subsided, Kevin decided to leave. We didn't think about it when he arrived at the hospital, but he had driven almost three hours in that storm just to check on Ryan's condition. After the storm had moved on to the east, he decided to leave. Another storm cell was forecasted to the western part of the state, the direction he was going later that evening and he did not want to make the return trip in the second storm. We had prayer together and Kevin left.

We stayed at the hospital all day long, but we didn't do a lot other than sit in the waiting room telling funny stories and enjoying one another's company. At one point that evening the receptionist was straightening the waiting room. We started regaling her with stories and she laughed until she was in tears. There were not many other people in and out of the waiting room during that time, so we were free to laugh and enjoy ourselves without making others feel uncomfortable. The atmosphere was vastly different from the first time in the PICU waiting area, and we all knew it. God had done amazing things in Ryan's life and we were so overjoyed that we could not be discouraged at all, not even about the little soldier being grumpy and not wanting us in the room.

We left the hospital a little before visiting hours ended. We actually were able to go out the front doors of the building, something that had seldom happened in November. Just before we headed down to the lobby to leave, I checked on Ryan one last time. I just stood in his room shaking my head as I realized how incredibly good he looked. He had one IV in his leg, in case there was an emergency and they could not access his port. He was wearing pajamas and he had minimal swelling to his head as a whole. His eyes were still swollen quite a lot, to the point he could not see. He was resting well, so we left the hospital with light hearts and went to the motel to get a decent night's rest.

I had made plans to be away from my church on Sunday, so I could be in Little Rock at least through the weekend. On Sunday morning, before we went to the hospital, I was feeling very grateful to God for all He had done in Ryan's life. I felt as if I would burst if I did not verbalize all of the feelings pent up inside of me, so I did what I often did when those feelings welled up inside of me. I began to journal. I had been scolded so many times about making people cry when they read my entries I felt that I needed to give a quick warning that this was a moving entry and would most likely bring tears. I had some people tell me when I warned about tears going to fall, they would put off reading the journal, until they were in a private place, or until a time that running mascara would not be a problem.

This journal update was extremely profound to me for some reason. I had written many entries, but this one really put things in perspective for me in a way I had not even considered. It became a rally cry for each and every one of us. I include the entry in its complete state to help give the mindset we all had following the surgery. The last line in the entry pretty much summed everything up in words, which to this day, still bring joy to my heart. I did edit the entry to remove the name of the neurosurgeon. I did not wish to publish the full name of any of the medical staff, because I could not foresee what ramifications such attention might bring. Dr. X is the head neurosurgeon who performed the second surgery on Ryan.

SUNDAY, FEBRUARY 25, 2007 08:16 AM, CST
Caution- Watch for falling tears.

I have been thinking about those four words a lot the past two days - "We got it all" and wondered what they really meant. Here is what I have come to realize.

We - The doctor is admitting that he did not do all of this by himself. There were other doctors and nurses in the OR, but I think that Dr. X realizes that even outside the OR people contributed to Ryan's successful surgery. Ryan's mother and father have held his hand and encouraged him comforted his fears and loved him unconditionally. Then there was the family around Chris and Andrea, who have supported Chris and Andrea through all of this. By family, I refer not only to those of us who are blood-related, but those who have prayed, encouraged, and given whatever they could in support. The collective We in the successful surgery is everyone who reads this journal, who prays, who encourages. From my perspective, anybody who wants to can step up, shout it from the rooftops "We got it all," and know they helped defeat this monster.

Got-OK, standing alone not the greatest usage of the English language, but it lets me know that control is on our side. It is within our grasp, not running freely to do whatever damage it wants. Possession is on the side of the victors, not on the side of the cancer.

It-That devil spawn from the very pits of hell -- Cancer. Dr. X did not mince words here. It is specifically the tumor, which was draining the very life from this precious child. "It," like the B-movie monster of old, "The Blob." "It" was an amorphous being, which had been growing. The growth was not beneficial in any way; actually, "It" was quite harmful. Left unchecked, it is lethal. All of the doctors agree, "It" would have killed Ryan if they hadn't done something. Well, "It" is no more; "It" is gone.

All-I think this word has lost its meaning in this materialist world. We seem to want it "All." Things keep changing, improvements are made on a continual basis, and we don't ever get it "all." Well in this case, improvements are not on the way, and when the doctor said "All," he meant exactly that. There is no cancer in Ryan's little head. He is battered and he is bruised. He is sore and a little bit grouchy. However, one thing he is not. He is not an owner of a disastrous tumor. It is "All" gone.

"We got it all" -- maybe it will come back, maybe it won't. There is nothing we can do to prevent it if it does. If it were to come back, we will do what we have to then. Don't borrow trouble from tomorrow for today. REJOICE, SING IT, SHOUT IT, PASS THE WORD -- WE GOT IT ALL and for now, that is enough. Uncle Tim.

Miracles Never Cease

Sunday was a day of rapid change for Ryan. After we arrived at the hospital, we again took turns to visit Ryan. When I entered the room, I walked into a firestorm fight.

"But I'm hungry. Can't I have something to eat?" Ryan begged.

"OK, I will allow you to have something LIGHT to eat," replied the charge nurse.

"Is catfish LIGHT food?" Ryan immediately shot back.

"No, catfish is not LIGHT food," retorted the nurse.

"How about sausage links, are they LIGHT food?" he pressed the issue.

"No, sausage links are not LIGHT food either," came the reply.

"Cheetos?" He continued down his want list.

"Yes, I will allow you to have some Cheetos if you want them," she finally relented.

I went to the vending machine, got him a bag of Cheetos, and rushed them back to him. He thought he was going to starve. He had not eaten since the meal at The Olive Garden on Thursday night. It was now nearing noon on Sunday. I guess he should have been hungry.

His eyes still remained swollen shut, so I opened the bag and handed him the Cheetos one after another. After a half-dozen or so, he stopped.

Perplexed as to why he quit, I asked him, "Why did you quit? Did you already get full?"

"No, but the crunching of the Cheetos is making my head hurt worse," he lamented.

After he had eaten those few Cheetos and they remained in his stomach, the decision was made to move him to the neurology ward on the fourth floor. The swelling in Ryan's head had started shifting downward and by early afternoon, he began to be able to see out of one of his eyes, however the other one was still swollen shut.

Shortly after Ryan was settled into his new room, Jenti and Shannon had left the hospital to return to Missouri. Andrea and Ashtyn had also left so they could return to Pea Ridge. Nonna, Poppa, Chris, and I remained at the hospital with Ryan. As evening approached, Chris decided it was time to get something to eat for himself. Once again, he decided he wanted a steak. He did not want the steak from Colton's Steakhouse this time though. He had found another steakhouse one day while he was driving around Little Rock. Poppa did not want a steak, and Nonna did not want to leave the hospital. I ended up settling the matter by taking Poppa with me to get something for the two of us. We ate and I took him to the motel to get some additional rest. I then stopped at the restaurant to get steak dinners for Chris and Nonna.

When I returned to the hospital, Chris was famished and Ryan was doing his best to convince someone to give him something to eat as well. Ryan ate part of Nonna's steak and part of Chris' baked potato. He munched the croutons off both salads and then he finished off the meal by eating the rest of his Cheetos. He had eaten well, but he paid the price for it.

By the time Ryan was finished eating, his head had started throbbing again. Once the pain set in, it increased exponentially. He lay there and began to whine. At first, he whined only a little, but then he began to become more vocal about wanting relief. Finally, he reached his crescendo by yelling, "I need morphine!" It was almost as if he was a little drug addict looking to score a fix. We wanted to help him, but there was nothing we could do. He had reached a similar level of pain a few hours earlier, shortly after being moved from the PICU. They had given him morphine then, and it was too soon after that dose to give him more. Actually, he had been receiving morphine since the surgery had been completed. He was most definitely aware of the pain reduction when the morphine was in his system and when it was not. After about forty-five minutes after the pain began to set in, the nurse said he could have more morphine.

The nurse gave him the morphine and in a few minutes, Ryan had drifted off to sleep. Knowing it could be a long night for Chris, Nonna and I left the hospital early to allow Chris to rest while Ryan was resting.

If you have read this far in this book, you have already read past the journal entry that I wrote on Thanksgiving Day, 2007. I would like you to go back to that entry and re-read it before you continue. I would like every reader to stop and think about what I had written in November and then read what had transpired from February 23 to February 25, 2007. I had said in that journal entry that I felt God had spoken to me and told me I should not be downhearted because He had not told me what the outcome of anything was going to be. As the events of these three days had unfolded, it became very clear God did indeed have a plan in Ryan's life. For a little boy who had spent the better part of eight days in a chemically induced coma following the first surgery,

Ryan had gone through surgery, PICU recovery, to a regular room and eating steak all within 48 hours.

Though the doctor was certain he had gotten the entire tumor, and we had taken that to heart, he decided Ryan would have an MRI on Monday to verify there were no hotspots on Ryan's brain. In order to perform the MRI, Ryan was once again NPO, starting at midnight Sunday. We knew he was scheduled to have the MRI on Monday morning, but we had no idea what kind of morning we were in for when we got to the hospital the next day.

Prior to the MRI, an NPO sign was posted on Ryan's door. When we entered the room on Monday morning, we were informed by Ryan that his room was an NPO room and that meant there was to be no food or drink for anyone in the room. Nonna and I each had a cup of coffee and Ryan informed us we could not drink them.

I sat down at the end of Ryan's bed and Nonna sat down on the couch along the wall. Ryan's one eye was still swollen mostly shut and the other he had closed most of the time. I thought I could quietly drink my coffee without incident. I was wrong. I bent down and picked up my coffee cup. I shielded the cup with my hand and I took a little sip of coffee.

Ryan said, "I know what you are doing; I can see the part of your cup sticking out from behind your arm. If you take another drink, you are going to have to find some other place to do it."

I tried to explain that coffee is not any good if it gets cold, and it should be drank while it was hot and fresh.

He informed me, "If it gets cold, you can just get some more later."

I was beaten. I put my cup down and did not try for another sip. Nonna, however, tried to be ever so sly. There were big windows in Ryan's room and they faced the courtyard outside. Nonna turned her back to Ryan and acted as if she was looking out into the courtyard. While she was turned around, she took a drink of coffee from her cup.

Ryan barked at her, "Nonna, I know what you're doing; you are not allowed to eat or drink in here if I can't."

Nonna put her cup down and did not try for another drink either.

The whole time, Chris had assumed the fetal position on the couch and acted as if a bear was attacking. He and Ryan had been going at it tooth and nail most of the night.

About noon, Chris loaded Ryan into one of the wagons that the hospital had and took him down to get his MRI. As soon as he awakened from his MRI, he was allowed to eat; and did he ever eat. He had pizza and chips when he awoke and then made plans for us to get him catfish for dinner.

I had begun to notice he was not complaining about pain the way he had complained on Sunday. I asked Chris about it and he told me Ryan had not had any morphine since the dose that was given before we left on Sunday night. He was taking Tylenol for the pain and had not complained the entire day about the pain. Within forty-eight hours of having his head laid open and the tumor removed, Ryan was taking Tylenol for the pain.

The MRI results were completed by early afternoon and the neurosurgeon took Chris and me down to view the results and explain them to us. He showed us the MRI and he told us it had confirmed the cancer was completely gone. He said if any stray cells remained, the continued chemotherapy would take care of them. He told us there was no blood supply to any cancer cells and as such, Ryan's cancer was gone. The tumor was gone; the doctor proclaimed it and the test confirmed it. We were ecstatic.

There was only one more thing to discuss with the doctor before we left the office. Ryan was bored and he wanted out of the bed. He told Chris to find out from the doctor when that could happen. Chris said he would ask the doctor, but it would probably be a while.

As we prepared to leave the doctor's office, Chris dutifully asked the doctor Ryan's question. The doctor looked a little surprised and thought it over for a minute. "I don't see any problem with him getting out of bed if he feels like it. I would like for one of the physical therapists to be present when he gets up the first time, just as a precaution."

We walked away from that meeting with the doctor and we felt as if we were walking on air. The doctor was completely convinced the cancer had been removed and Ryan was going to be getting out of bed to walk around within 72 hours of the surgery. It completely floored us when the doctor told us Ryan could get out of bed, but at the same time it really was just another answer to all of the prayers that had been prayed on Ryan's behalf in the weeks leading up to the surgery.

Ryan was very anxious to get out of bed, but Chris told him he had to wait until the therapist could get there. Since Ryan was on the neurology ward and not on the therapy ward, it took several hours for someone to get to him. While we waited for a therapist to get to Ryan, we decided it would be a good time to get Ryan's catfish. Catfish sounded tasty to all of us, so Chris, Poppa, and I all went to a restaurant to eat catfish and when we got finished we took some back to Ryan. He did not like the fish, it was too cold and not to his liking. He grumbled and complained about it and decided to eat his food from the hospital. Chris told him they would get some of the catfish he liked at the end of the week and that appeased Ryan somewhat.

Shortly after we returned from dinner, one of the therapists was able to get to Ryan. I stood in the hall so there was enough space to move around in Ryan's room. I started taking pictures: first was Ryan standing, then there was Ryan taking a step, and then Ryan after he had walked out of his room into the hall. He stopped in the hall and posed for a picture for me. He was weak and a little unstable, but he was up and walking under his own control.

When he had walked into the hall and back, Ryan got back into his bed and just sat looking very pleased with himself. In just over 72 hours Ryan was not only standing up, he walked from his bed into the hallway, walked around the hall a few minutes, and then walked back to his room. The whole time he had a hand to help steady himself, but the hand was simply there to steady him, nothing more.

After Ryan got back into his bed, he worked on a craft project the therapist had given him. It was a fun project for him because the therapist wanted him to make some animals. She gave him several latex gloves and some markers. We inflated the gloves for Ryan and he created all types of animals by tying them together and decorating them with the markers. When he got finished with his craft, he got his coloring book and colors back out and colored for a while. He was a totally different child than he had been twenty-four hours earlier, when he had been screaming that he needed morphine. It was almost as if sometime during the previous night, he was miraculously touched and his pain removed.

We stayed until it was time for visiting hours to be over and then we headed back to the motel. The next morning Poppa and I planned to leave Little Rock and head home. We were going to leave Nonna and Poppa's car in Little Rock, so Chris could drive anywhere he might need to go during the week. Andrea had returned to Pea Ridge in their van and she could not return until Friday after Ashtyn finished school for the week. We hadn't been given any solid idea of when Ryan would get out of the hospital, but the plan was if he got out of the hospital before Friday, Chris, Nonna, and Ryan would drive to Searcy and stay at Carnell's house. Andrea would meet them in Searcy rather than Little Rock and Nonna could make the trip from Searcy to Poplar Bluff. She did not want to drive in Little Rock traffic, but she felt that she could handle the trip from Searcy on her own, when the time came. We were not sure when Ryan would be released, but due to the distances everyone had to travel, we felt it best to have a travel plan in place before everyone went their separate ways.

Nonna moved her suitcase into the RMH the day that Andrea left for Pea Ridge. Chris had the room reserved and either he or Nonna would use the room to have a place to sleep while the other one stayed in the hospital room with Ryan. On Tuesday morning, Poppa and I checked out of the motel and went to the hospital about the time visiting hours started so we could check in on Ryan and then get on the road as quickly as possible. On the way to the hospital, we went and bought doughnuts. Ryan had asked us to bring doughnuts since he was not going to be NPO when we got there that morning.

Ryan's surgery had been on February 23, and when I prepared to leave the hospital on February 27, I was stunned at the progress he had made. He had already had his port de-accessed, which meant he was finished with the IV. The therapist had visited his room before we got to the hospital that morning. She was still in the room working with Ryan when we arrived. She was helping him walk around when we entered the room with the doughnuts. He walked around the bed to the couch where Nonna was sitting, climbed up onto the couch, and helped himself to a big Bavarian Crème doughnut.

His mental acuity was a joy to witness. I was playing a joke on him, or so I thought, and I asked him the question, "If you have one goose and two geese, what do you have if you have two moose?"

I expected the common answer that you would have two "meese," or perhaps two "mooses."

"If you had two moose, you would have a deuce, silly."

I was not anticipating his response and I burst into laughter. I realized at that point that he was mentally sharper than I was and I changed the conversation.

The therapist told us that morning that Ryan's left side was stronger than it had been when he left the hospital in January. Since she had been his therapist in January also, she knew what level of performance he had achieved by then. Her proclamation meant Ryan had not lost any of his motor skills due to the surgery and his progress had not been impeded. From a therapy standpoint, he was right where he had been the previous Thursday before the surgery. The main difference was he did not have cancer any longer.

With that incredible piece of information, Poppa and I left the hospital and headed toward his house. We made it as far as Searcy before we stopped to get fuel. As I was fueling the van, my phone rang.

The caller ID said that it was Chris. I answered the phone and heard him laughing on the other end. I thought he was going to tell me something funny Ryan had said or done.

"What is it with you?" he cackled.

"I don't think I want to answer that without a bit more to the question?" I wittily replied.

"The doctor just left Ryan's room and he told us Ryan will be released from the hospital in the morning. If you had stuck around one more day, you would have gotten to be here when he was released."

"I don't know why he keeps doing that to me. I guess next time I will just plan a shorter stay and everyone else will benefit from that," I bemoaned.

I left Little Rock once; Ryan woke up from his chemical coma. I left a second time; Ryan started walking and riding the tricycle. I left the third time; and Ryan had progressed so well he would be out of the hospital in a matter of days following his second surgery. I had missed witnessing all of those major events, but at least he was making huge strides to get better, so I couldn't complain much.

Poppa and I continued toward home, but we had much lighter hearts than before, knowing Ryan would be released from the hospital the next morning. We talked about going back and spending one more night in Little Rock, but I had arranged my schedule to be home on Tuesday night and I had things I needed to do there. We also would be running the risk that we had stayed without a valid reason if Ryan had not been released the next morning. We decided it was best to follow the plan we had created originally.

As Poppa and I talked on the way to his house, we were just in awe about how good God had been. We conferred and decided it had to have been the prayer support before the surgery that caused such a drastic difference in the recovery process. I believe God was just giving us a taste of His awesome power and letting us know there was nothing He couldn't accomplish.

I dropped Poppa off at his house and I headed to my house. I made it home late on Tuesday night. The next morning right on schedule, Ryan was released from the hospital. Knowing Ryan was supposed to be released was great news, but to find out he had been officially released was such a lift. We had church the night he was released and I was thrilled to share with them from the time we had met the previous Wednesday night, Ryan had already had his surgery and had been released from the hospital.

We were not so thrilled with what happened following Ryan's release from the hospital though. I phoned Chris on Thursday to see how Ryan had done after his release. He filled me in on what had happened through the night.

Ryan had developed a fever so Chris had taken him to the emergency room in Searcy. The ER staff had done their best to care for him. They gave him Tylenol and Motrin to bring the fever down and then they had sent him home for the night. The morning dawned with Ryan still battling the fever, so Chris called the hospital in Little Rock for guidance. The doctors quickly conferred and told Chris that Ryan needed to return to the hospital in Little Rock. Thursday morning Chris and Nonna returned to Little Rock and Ryan was re-admitted to the hospital.

The doctors did not have any good reasons for why Ryan had spiked the fever. His blood work showed no sign of infection. There was concern that the shunt in Ryan's head could be causing the problem. The doctors speculated there could be some kind of infection in the fluid that the shunt drained. So, some of the fluid was collected to test. The test they performed was for meningitis, which could be deadly if that was the cause of the fever. This was not a quick test, as a culture had to be grown. Chris did not want people to panic over the possibility that Ryan might have meningitis, so that information was not made public outside of the family. As the day passed on Thursday, the doctors worked feverishly to keep Ryan's temperature down and to try to find the cause of the fever.

The battle to keep Ryan's body temperature normal was waged all night long that Thursday night. I spoke with Chris on Friday and all was pretty much as it had been the day before. The doctors could not find a source of infection. The blood work did not show any signs of abnormality. The cultures they were growing had to grow for forty-eight hours and the results would not be ready until Saturday. All that could be done was to alternate Motrin and Tylenol in an attempt to regulate his temperature.

The culture results were given on Saturday and everything was fine with them. Ryan did not have an infection in his spinal fluid. The doctors could only speculate Ryan had a virus and with the thousands of viruses in the world, they could only tell Chris which viruses Ryan did not have. The cultures they had done eliminated the most severe viruses by having a negative result. Cultures only showed if a particular virus was present. If the virus was present, it would grow in the culture dish. If the virus was not present, the culture dish remained empty. The only way to confirm a particular virus was to try to grow that particular virus. With thousands of choices, doctors only grew cultures for the more lethal varieties. Based on the cultures that had been grown, Ryan did not have any of those varieties.

After struggling to determine the cause of the fever from Thursday until the culture results were known on Saturday afternoon, the doctors decided it must be a virus and so they stopped pursuing a cause and conceded that the best they could do was treat the fever to keep it down. Ironically, within a few hours of getting the culture results, the fever disappeared on its own. When it was time for the next dose of Motrin, Ryan's temperature was normal. The doctor decided to withhold the medicine until his fever started elevating once more. It never rose again. On Sunday, after he had been fever free for over twelve hours, Ryan was released and allowed to return to Carnell's house in Searcy. He could have gone home to Pea Ridge, but he had a check-up with the neurologist on Tuesday, so they stayed in Searcy so he would have a shorter trip to the hospital on Tuesday.

The doctor's appointment on Tuesday, March 6, 2007, was a day that was marked on the calendar with great importance. The doctor's who had performed the second surgery saw Ryan and determined there was no longer any reason for him to remain a neurology patient and they officially released him as a neurology patient. His case was transferred to the Hematology/Oncology Department. The stitches from his surgery were removed and Ryan was allowed to go home. Ryan would begin having his steroids removed from his medications, but this time it would be much more gradual than the first attempt.

It was about this time that it began to gel with me that God was instructing me to write this book. As I wrote about the various acts, they began to evolve in my mind as the separate sections of the book. I did not tell anyone of this idea at first because I did not want to write a book. I did not know how to write a book and above everything else, I really did not have the time to write a book. Ryan's tumor was gone, he was doing well, and he was settling back into a normal life for a little boy. I really thought that the whole ordeal was nearing completion. Little did I know.

Once Ryan was released from the neurology department, the family went home to Pea Ridge. I did not pester them on a daily basis, but I did keep up with how Ryan was doing on a frequent basis. When I would speak to Chris, it was clear Ryan was settling into his routine. He was working on his schoolwork and life was going great.

Ryan continued to progress astoundingly well from his hospital release until the middle of March, and on March 14, Ryan began his first round of home based chemotherapy. It did not go so well. The level of chemotherapy medicine they prescribed for Ryan as a maintenance dose was over two times the amount he had taken during the days in Little Rock. He became very ill and could not keep food down for several days during the treatment.

It was very difficult for Chris and Andrea to see Ryan so sick as he took the chemo. He had done so well the first time they expected similar results this time. The increased dosage was just more than his little body could withstand. It made him very sick and caused him to be extremely fatigued. The concerns were forwarded to the doctors in Little Rock, and their response was to prescribe a stronger anti-nausea medicine. This new medicine was to be in addition to the anti-nausea medicine Ryan was already taking.

Ryan finished his chemotherapy on a Sunday night. The home health care nurse came on Monday to draw blood for evaluation. During the days that he could not stand to eat, Ryan had been drinking Gatorade to try to keep his electrolytes where they needed to be. The blood work showed his potassium level had dropped drastically due to him having been so sick from the chemotherapy. If the potassium level had dropped any lower, he would have been admitted to the hospital, but as it turned out, he started to rebound before it caused him to be admitted. It was on Thursday following the completion of that round of chemotherapy that Ryan was finally able to take food into his system and not get sick.

One very exciting thing occurred during the time Ryan was taking the first round of maintenance chemotherapy. He was notified he had been accepted to play on a T-ball team, the Fighting Frogs. He had asked early on if he could play and the doctors had told Chris and Andrea if he felt like playing, it would be a good source of therapy for him. They had signed him up and during that week of chemotherapy, he found out he had been placed on the team. Though he was weak from the chemotherapy, he was extremely excited about getting on a T-ball team.

Me, I was awestruck about him being placed on a T-ball team. Here was a precious child, who had lain in a chemically induced coma less than five months before, who had been through an eight-plus hour surgery less than one month before, defeating the odds and being placed on a T-ball team. God had granted Ryan an incredible strength to see him through the surgeries, but here was Ryan going so far above surviving that it boggled the mind. God had performed yet another miracle. Ryan had not only survived, he had thrived. We had prayed for God to preserve Ryan's life. God had other plans yet again. Not only was Ryan to survive, he was to excel and show the world the power of God. We had the blessing of being able to share that miracle with anyone who would listen.

Victory!

My wife had to go to San Francisco the third week of March 2007, and I had the opportunity to go with her. We flew out on Sunday, March 18, and flew back on Saturday, March 24. During this whole time, Ryan was fighting the effects of the chemo. Nonna had come to our house to stay with my kids while we were gone to San Francisco. As he struggled with the side effects of the chemotherapy through the week, we were not sure whether or not they would end up in Little Rock with the poor little guy.

As difficult as that round of chemo was, Ryan did make it through and he began to get stronger toward the end of the week. As we were returning from San Francisco, Ryan was back on his feet again. I think it could have been the excitement about T-ball practice that spurred him onward. He was so excited to be on a team and he looked forward to getting to play. As he was recovering from his chemotherapy, practices were just beginning. He was able to participate in his first practice just before spring break.

The school that Ashtyn and Ryan attended had spring break the last week of March. With that knowledge in mind, the next round of check-ups for Ryan had been scheduled at the beginning of that week. On March 26, Ryan had to go to the hematology/oncology clinic and have his blood tested. Following his check-up, the family would head northward and visit Nonna and Poppa's house in Missouri, where they would spend the remainder of spring break. The timing of all of the events allowed Laura and I to return home just in time for Nonna to go home and prepare for her guests.

I had mistakenly thought Ryan only had one check-up in Little Rock, but I found it was actually multiple check-ups that had been scheduled for the same day. Ryan spent most of the day in the hospital. All of his blood counts were acceptable, except for the potassium level. It had never rebounded completely from the week of chemotherapy. As I spoke with Chris, he was in transit to meet Andrea, so we talked about the results while he drove.

"The doctor told Ryan he had a solution to help with getting the potassium level elevated. He said that Gatorade does an okay job of replenishing electrolytes, but when a patient's potassium level gets as low as Ryan's, it is not enough. Bananas are a good source of potassium, and so are a lot of other food sources. He had one item though that he thought Ryan might like a little better. The doctor said Gatorade was processed by the body as a liquid. His alternative supplement has proteins and fat that encapsulates potassium and cause the body to slow down metabolism. This gives the potassium more of a chance to absorb into the body."

"I am with you so far," I said. "What is the supplement?"

Laughing like a hyena, Chris responded, "Yoo-Hoo chocolate drink."

"What is so funny about that?" I wondered aloud.

"It just seems very funny to me that a doctor is telling Ryan that he needs to drink a sugary sweet chocolate drink to help combat the effects of chemotherapy. It just doesn't seem like a normal thing for a doctor to prescribe," Chris continued, "but then nothing else about Ryan's case has been normal has it?"

"You're right about that," I concluded.

We talked for a few more minutes, about what they had plans to do during the remaining days of spring break.

Chris stopped laughing finally, "Seriously though, the doctor is concerned about the toll that the last round of chemotherapy took on Ryan. He doesn't want to decrease the level of that medicine though. He reiterated the aggressive nature of the cancer that Ryan had and he does not want to give it a chance to gain a foothold and re-form. He wants to continue blasting any stray cancer cells with the maximum chemotherapy dosage possible. He gave me a prescription for a new, more powerful, anti-nausea medicine. We are to try that and see if Ryan can tolerate that much chemotherapy in conjunction with the new anti-nausea medicine. If it does work, great, if that combination doesn't work, we are going to talk about where to go during the next doctor's appointment."

"So what else is happening with Ryan, is his hair starting to return yet?" I asked.

"Yeah, it is coming back, but it is very uneven still. I am keeping it cut extra short. I am still keeping my head shaved also. I am sure glad spring is almost here. My head has been cold all winter. Did I tell you about Ryan's brace?" Chris paused.

"I know he has been wearing one. Did they change that during the doctor's visit?"

"Not exactly," Chris began again. "During T-ball practice last week he fell and broke his brace."

"He fell! Is he okay?" I interjected.

"Hang on a second and let me explain," Chris replied. "He had been off the chemotherapy for about four days, but he was still a little weak from being so sick. He went to practice even though he was weak and he was extremely glad to be there. He was up to bat and he hit the ball. He tossed the bat down and started toward first base. He can't run yet, so he was quick-walking as fast as he could. He didn't see the bat in his way in time to avoid it and he tripped over it. Since he was so weak, he couldn't keep himself from falling. Down he went. I am not sure how it happened, but during the fall, he broke his brace. We have to get it fixed, but it will take a little while before they can get it done. The doctor said Ryan could wear high-top tennis shoes for now, but he has to take it slow so he doesn't turn his ankle. Other than the broken brace, the fall didn't hurt him."

"So are you going to let him keep playing? What happens if he falls again? He could get hurt much worse."

"Well, we talked to his coach, who is also the league president, and he gave us permission to have me run alongside Ryan to help keep that from happening again. I am going to hold onto his hand and keep him stable. I can kick the bat out of the way if that sort of thing happens again," came Chris' reply.

"How do the other parents and coaches feel about that?" I pushed a little further.

"The parents in the stands started crying when he fell and started cheering when he picked himself up and continued on to first base. He was out by the time he got there and as he walked off the field, they gave him a standing ovation. He did cry a little when he got back to the dugout, but he was okay. The parents don't have a problem and the other coaches don't seem to have a problem either. It wouldn't matter if they didn't let me hold onto his hand anyhow. I would not make him stop playing. He loves it so much I could not take that joy away from him. It would break his heart if we said he couldn't play now. No, I will protect him as much as possible, but I won't break his heart to protect his body. He will be fine to play. I hope you can come and see him play at least one game. Hey, it's been great talking with you, but I have to go now. I am meeting with Andrea and we are headed on towards Mom and Dad's house. I will talk with you later," and Chris hung up.

After they met, Chris, Andrea, and the kids headed for Nonna and Poppa's house. They arrived safely and then the "break" began in earnest. Many people had been following Ryan's case on the website. When word hit the website that Ryan was going to be at Nonna and

Poppa's house, phone calls started to flood their house. One person after another called to ask if it would be okay for them to stop and see Ryan. Instead of trying to limit the number of people who were going to be at the house, Nonna invited them all to come. She and Chris discussed the situation and decided that rather than have people coming in every day, it would be better if they would all show up at one time. They decided to hold an open house and cook dinner for anyone who wanted to show up at the house.

The house Nonna and Poppa live in used to be a restaurant and when the business closed, they converted the entire building into a home. At one point, there was seating for roughly 150. That was a very structured setting with diner tables and chairs. Since it had been converted, there was much less seating room. The kitchen, however, was more than adequate to prepare a huge meal. One of the gifts that Nonna possesses is a gift of hospitality. Anyone is welcome to drop in and there is always food around. The plan was simple: cook lots, invite whoever wanted to come, and enjoy the evening.

I really wanted to attend the open house, but having just gotten back from San Francisco and getting ready for another trip, I couldn't fit it in. The second trip was going to make up for it anyhow. The first week of April was the week my kids all had spring break. We had talked it over with Chris and Andrea and decided that we would all go to their house the following week, during our spring break. Our plan was to go to Chris and Andrea's house the first part of the week and then go to my in-laws home toward the end of the week. My in-laws lived about 40 miles from Nonna and Poppa, so we planned on stopping by Nonna and Poppa's on the way back to our home. We were going to make a big circle across Missouri into northwest Arkansas, then circle back across southeast Missouri, and finally return to Illinois. When Ryan found out we were going to be at Nonna's the next week he decided he would just stay there so he could see our family. When they told him he couldn't do that he became rather put out with everyone. They did not want to tell him we were going to be at his house; that was a surprise for him. Fortunately, the open house at Nonna's came along and got Ryan's mind off the fact we were not there.

The night of the open house, Nonna and Chris started cooking early. They fixed fried chicken, French fries, ham, corn, green beans and cottage cheese, plus desserts. Before the end of the night, more than thirty people came to visit Ryan. It was a very enjoyable night for all involved.

After hearing about the success of the open house at Nonna's house, I called Chris and talked to him about having an open house the following week, when we were at his house. We decided to go to The Olive Garden, commonly referred to as "The OG" by Ryan, in Fayetteville. I wrote an update for the website to announce the date and time we were going to be at the restaurant. We invited anyone who wanted to meet Ryan to drop by that evening.

Ryan had a great time at Nonna and Poppa's house. He even got to go fishing. Grandpa Roscoe (Poppa's dad), Poppa, Chris, and Ryan all went fishing together, four generations on a fishing trip. What a great picture that would have been, but unfortunately Chris didn't have anyone to take the picture with him in it. He took a picture of Grandpa Roscoe, Poppa, and Ryan fishing. We included that photo on the website and it received rave reviews from the site readers. Ryan looked so happy being outside, fishing with his grandpa and great-grandpa.

As the week ended, everyone was saddened that it was almost over. It had been a great deal of fun for everyone. The guests at the open house were all amazed at how great Ryan looked. It was a huge blessing for all of those people who had been praying for Ryan to get to witness firsthand the miracles that God had performed in his life.

The time had come for Chris and Andrea to head home. They had to get home and prepare for our arrival the next Monday. We on the other hand finished wrapping everything up so we could make our trip.

Monday morning rolled around and we started on our journey. While we were en route to Chris' house, Chris found out that a friend of Ryan's from ACH, was back in the hospital. While Ryan was out and about on his spring break trip, his friend had taken a turn for the worse and she was admitted back into ACH. Her condition continued to worsen and Chris sent out a request for prayer for her. The doctors told the family if they wanted to say goodbye to her, they needed to come to ACH and do so. It was not expected for her to survive the week. However, God is good. In a matter of days, God had intervened in her life and she began to get better.

We made it to the house Monday evening early and spent that night just having a good time. Around 10:00 p.m., everyone, except Chris and I, had headed for bed. We decided to go outside and sit on the deck so we could talk. While we talked, I decided to reveal to him that I was working on this book.

"I don't really know how to explain this, but here goes," I began. "I have been feeling like God has been guiding me to write a book about

Ryan's life. I have tried to shake the feeling, but it won't go away. It feels like God has his thumb in my back, pushing me to write it."

Chris contemplated that for a moment, "So how is it going?"

"I believe I should start with the day he was diagnosed and tell the story from that point forward. Here is the thing. I don't want to write a book, sell it, and make money because of the suffering that Ryan has had to undergo. I don't know how to handle the financial aspect of the whole situation. I believe I should write, but then I don't know what to do."

"I can see your dilemma," came his reply.

"It is my book, but it is about your son," I continued. "First off, how do you feel about me writing about him?"

"I think it is an awesome idea. God has brought him through so much that his story needs to be told. I think you would be the perfect one to write the story." He hesitated and then continued, "What if we donated part of the profits, a tenth of the profit to the church, then a portion of the profit to the Children's Miracle Network, and then put money back for all of the kids for college."

"Works for me," I momentarily paused, then continued, "I didn't know how to address this whole discussion. I didn't want money to become a stumbling block between us. I think we are on the same page about the financial part now. I feel much better about the whole situation. Now all I have to do is get busy writing."

We talked until after 2:00 in the morning about the outline of the book and I clarified some details about which I was a little fuzzy. Finally, we became so tired we had to go to bed. I went to bed that night with a huge burden lifted. I had dreaded discussing the financial factors involved with writing this book, but we had worked through all of the details and reached a great conclusion I felt. It was clearer to me than ever before, God wanted me to chronicle Ryan's life to share the miracles He had performed on Ryan's behalf.

The next day when we got up, Chris and I went to his garage where he had a small woodworking shop set up. In his spare time, he made ink pens from exotic woods. He showed me how to make one, and then we spent the better part of the day taking turns making ink pens. With their spring break being over, Ashtyn and Ryan had returned to their normal routines. Ashtyn had to go to school and Ryan had therapy during the day. Andrea took my daughter, Rebekah, for lunch with Ashtyn. They bought meals and went to the school where the three of them were able to eat together. After lunch, Ryan had to go to therapy, so my daughter, Jessica, went with Andrea and Ryan to the therapy session. Ryan really enjoyed showing off for Jessica during therapy. Joshua had to work that week, so he did not get to make the trip with us. He missed being with us, but it couldn't be helped.

That evening for dinner, we went to "The OG" for the open house. We did not have as large of a gathering as they had at Nonna's the week before, be we still had almost twenty people show up that night to meet Ryan. Again, the visitors that came were astounded by how good Ryan looked. Those that had been following his case were overwhelmed at the goodness of God. Throughout the evening, tears were continually shed as we relived some of the events of the previous months. As people shared how they had heard about Ryan, our hearts were filled with gratitude because of their compassion. We enjoyed a great meal that evening, and we grew better acquainted with some of the prayer warriors who had helped us wage the battle that was Ryan's life.

The morning after the open house, Laura, Jessica, Rebekah, and I started making the trip, which would eventually lead us home at the end of spring break. Our plan was followed without interruption and we returned home at the end of the week thoroughly worn out from all of the travel. Our lives finally were getting back to normal. During my trip to San Francisco and then the subsequent spring break trip, I had not gotten to work on this book. I settled back in and began to write.

Following the spring break trips for everyone, it was time for Ryan to have his next round of chemotherapy. There was a lot of concern about how he would handle the chemotherapy, but the doctors had given them the new prescription for anti-nausea medicine, so the hope was he would do well. The second round of chemotherapy went smoother for Ryan, he was able to keep his food down, and he was able keep his activity level as it was because the chemotherapy did not drain him as badly.

God had been so faithful once again. Not only had Ryan come through his chemotherapy much easier than the previous time, but also Ryan's friend had gotten to go home again. She had been to the doorstep of death and God had returned her to strength. It was becoming clear prayer is not some mystical solution where special words were uttered and God magically fixed everything. Prayer being offered caused us all to realize the extent to which we needed to rely on God for His strength and His provision.

I was thrilled when I found out Ryan's friend was home. She was also quite a fighter. I did not know her very well, I had met her in Little Rock, but I did not get to spend time with her or her family as Chris did. He was pretty close to the family and it really hurt him to see Ryan's friend go from remission to active leukemia. It signaled the reality that even if Ryan's cancer was gone, it could come back at any time. That was difficult, but I believe it was something that we all needed to accept. Ryan's cancer was gone but it could come back. All we could do was continue to pray about the situation and let God do the rest.

It was difficult to imagine that just a few months before we were journaling every day, and some days multiple times. As life became more active and continued to normalize, it just did not seem that journal updates were merited. There were only so many times you could put on the website that Ryan had his teacher come to the house and work on his school work with him. We could have sprinkled that information with the daily visits to therapy. T-ball practice was something that could be written about, but that only seemed interesting if there was a big play or a problem.

Take a moment to reflect on your own life. Did anything happen today that would merit a website update? Maybe there was and maybe there was not. That is what normal life is like. Some days are noteworthy, but it seems as if most days pass without notable highs or lows. Those days are the days we were experiencing in our lives and we loved every one of them. We had been to the deepest valleys on those days when Ryan was at his most critical. We had been to the highest mountaintops on days such as the day the doctor told us he had gotten the entire tumor. God had seen us through the good and the bad, and now we were satisfied in knowing He was walking hand in hand with us through these days when life was "normal."

The month of April passed with very little excitement. Ryan continued in his schoolwork, his blood work remained strong and his hair returned in fine form. Everyone was anxiously awaiting the season opener for the Fighting Frogs. However, the weather was not cooperative, and it rained out the season opener.

One of Ryan's schoolmates had a different form of cancer. This child was also on the Fighting Frogs team with Ryan. The child had been treated and was doing outstanding. It was amazing that in a town as small as Pea Ridge, there were two little boys who had overcome cancer. One thing that happened when people went through a situation like Ryan's, they began to find out they were not alone. The network of people who are caregivers to children with cancer is actually much larger than one might think. Once Chris found out about one of these children, he would keep in touch with their caregivers and track how the child was doing. At this time of the year, all of the children Chris checked on were doing well, even the one the doctors did not think would survive just a few weeks earlier.

Finally, on April 26, Ryan was able to play in his first T-ball game. Chris wrote the following entry for Ryan's website. I read the update and I wept once again, which was something that hardly ever happened before Ryan was diagnosed. The image of Ryan playing T-ball seemed surreal when I thought back to the horrible days of the previous November when Ryan could not even breathe on his own. To read the update was to stand humbled in the presence of God.

THURSDAY, APRIL 26, 2007 09:09 PM, CDT

The weather was cold and windy, the clouds were grey and rolling, and there was a very good chance the game would be rained out. Ryan and family got to the park and started warming up. Everyone was ready to play because it was so cold, but we had to wait until 6:30 p.m. At that time, the Fighting Frogs lined up on the third base line, removed their hats, and said the Pledge of Allegiance to the Flag. Lets Play Ball!!!! The Frogs were the visiting team and Ryan was first to bat. He hit the ball, but dragging dad down the baseline took too much time and he was out at first. He told me I had to run faster next time so they wouldn't get him out. The Frogs scored six runs in the first and so did the other team, the Cardinals. When Ryan got up to bat the next time, I told him I would run faster and I did. A hard hit to third and we were safe at first without even a throw. Both stands were so excited. We made it to second and then to third. One of the Frogs power hitters was up, he hit it to the outfield, and Ryan was able to SCORE!!! More heroic than when Kirk Gibson hit the homerun in the bottom of the 9th in the world series for the Dodgers, more awesome than an unassisted triple play, more impressive than Michael Jordan's 6 Championship rings, Ryan SCORED!!! Both stands cheered, tears flowed, the clouds started to clear and the sun came out. The next inning, more was wanted, but Ryan had a little stumble going to first and could not beat out the throw. The Frogs won the hard fought game, 15 to 12. I have added some new pictures of Ryan in uniform and one of the team and one of him and one of his best buddies. What started out to be a rainy, cloudy, windy, and cold game, ended with the

clouds parting and the beautiful sun setting. This game
was symbolic of Ryan's ordeal when it started. It was full
of gloom, but with God's help, it ended with a beautiful
sunset. I know we still have a long way to go, but Ryan
SCORED!!! More updates later. Dad

It had been an incredible lift to the spirits of our entire family when Ryan had been placed on a T-ball team and when he was able to go to practice, that was a highlight in our days. It was such a blessing to know even when he had been so weak from his chemotherapy, he had been able to power through so he could practice. His first game was huge though. He had not only been on a team and allowed to practice, he had actually played and he had scored. He had not only been playing, he had contributed to the winning of the game. His only assistance was from his dad steadying him as he made his way around the bases.

Chris noted Ryan had stumbled on his way to first base. As a result of stumbling, he was thrown out on the play to first base. As I spoke with Chris about his journal entry later that night, he told me he had to make a quick decision about that play.

"Ryan hit the ball down the third base line and off we went toward first base. Ryan stumbled for a moment and I stopped to steady him. I had to make a quick decision about that play. If I had kept going and steadying him at the same time, I could have helped him get to the base in time to be called safe. I didn't think that was fair though, so I stopped and let Ryan right himself before we went on to first. I didn't think it would be fair to give him an edge, so I let him do it on his own and he was out. I just kept him from falling."

"I think you made the right decision," I commented.

If someone was new to Ryan's website, they might have felt this was a very overly dramatic account of the game. It was a dramatic event though. Here was just another example of how glorious God was. He had not only allowed us to keep Ryan, He had blessed us with the ability to witness yet another miracle in the life of Ryan. To some people it was just a T-ball game, but to our family it was a milestone we did not know would ever happen.

Chris and Andrea were kept very busy for the next weeks with T-ball and softball practices and games. With Ryan and Ashtyn both playing, there was either a practice or a game almost every day. As the days passed, I talked with Chris on a routine basis. He never complained about the busyness of the situation. He was so blessed to have both of his children strong enough to play that he wouldn't dare make negative comments about it. They were wonderfully blessed and they knew it.

The first week of May arrived. In the midst of normalcy, there continued to be the need for doctor's visits. No matter how well Ryan appeared to be doing, he still had to go back to the doctors about once a month to be checked over. He had been playing ball and doing his therapy. He had been doing his schoolwork and having a great time being a little boy. It was now time for another doctor's visit and we did not know what to expect. It had been six months since this ordeal had begun. We were all very excited about his ability to play T-ball, but we could not see what was going on inside of his head or inside the rest of his body. When Ryan went for his May check-up, we found that all was not as well as we had hoped. He had been doing well from all external appearances, but during the check-up, we found out some information that we could not have known without the tests.

The follow-up visit on May 7, included an MRI. It had been six full months since Ryan had been diagnosed with the tumor. The results of the MRI indicated that the tumor was indeed completely gone. However, his blood work showed some problems. The tests showed that Ryan was neutropenic, which meant his white blood cell count was low. This occurred because of the chemotherapy and it caused a weakening of his immune system. The only way the body could build the white blood cells was by giving the body time to rebuild the cells. After he had been diagnosed as being neutropenic, Ryan had to begin wearing a mask over his mouth and nose when he was in public. He had to refrain from being indoors with groups of people. Indoors, people are generally in closer proximity to one another than outdoors. The doctor said Ryan could continue playing T-ball, but he needed to refrain from being indoors with groups. This would help reduce the risk of illness while his body was rebuilding the white blood cells.

Following his appointment at the hematology/oncology clinic, Ryan had one extra doctor's appointment when he went to Little Rock in May. He visited an optometrist to have his eyes checked. During that check-up, it was determined the tumor and the radiation had both been endured without damage to Ryan's eyes. His vision was perfectly normal for a little boy of six.

Ryan returned home to Pea Ridge that night, and the reports had been mostly positive. The neutropenia had concerned the doctor, so he decided to re-evaluate the situation before the next round of chemotherapy was under way.

Life back in Pea Ridge was in full swing and on May 10, Ryan was able to go to the school and have his Kindergarten graduation picture taken. Even with all of the time Ryan spent in the hospital and the Ronald McDonald House, he passed all of the tests that were required for him to be promoted to the first grade. He passed every subject with flying colors. Ryan would graduate Kindergarten, and he would participate in the graduation ceremony on June 1, 2007.

On the day of May 10, Mrs. Kennemer, Ryan's teacher, received a surprise presentation. Chris had nominated her for the Wal-Mart Teacher of the Year award. Each store honored a special teacher and she was chosen as the honoree for Store 100 in Bentonville, Arkansas. Ryan had to leave before the presentation, due to the neutropenia, but he heard all about the ceremony and he was thrilled for her.

After we knew that Ryan was going to be promoted to the first grade, the family discussed Ryan's graduation ceremony. We agreed we all wanted to witness the event, so Nonna, Poppa, Jenti and I all made plans to congregate in Pea Ridge and watch Ryan walk with his graduating class.

Friday, May 18, brought with it a new twist. Hulk Hogan was at Chris' office building to visit. Chris and his family, including his brother-in-law who had recently returned from Iraqi, went to the office to try to meet Mr. Hogan. The line was very long and they could not wait, so Chris went toward the head of the line to see if he knew anyone who would get some autographs for Ryan and Ashtyn. When he was walking around, Ryan was sitting on his shoulders and everyone started cheering for Ryan as they saw him. The crowd insisted that Chris take Ryan to the front of the line. Chris declined and told them the rest of his family was all toward the back of the line. He gracefully left the front-end of the line and headed back to his spot. Shortly after he was in his place, one of the representatives of the company went to him and told him the people in line had requested she get him and the rest of his family to go to the front of the line to meet Mr. Hogan. They had all gone to the front of the line and met the Hulkster. Ryan had his picture taken as he showed his "guns" (biceps) to Mr. Hogan. A camera crew was video taping the event, in case they chose to air the footage on the TV show "Hogan Knows Best." Chris had to sign a release, giving permission for the footage to be shown on TV. As far as we know, the footage never made it to TV. I wonder, if Mr. Hogan had heard Ryan's story, if he would have included the footage in his show. It didn't matter the footage didn't make it to TV. Ryan had met Mr. Hogan and had gotten his autograph. That was enough for him to be very excited.

As Ryan's graduation was approaching, my son Joshua graduated from high school. Nonna and Poppa made the trip to see their oldest grandson graduate from high school and my in-laws also made the trip to see Joshua graduate. With Ryan's rapidly approaching graduation on the horizon, Chris and Andrea did not try to squeeze a trip in to witness Joshua's graduation.

Ryan was scheduled to have the next round of chemotherapy the last week of May. As the date for the May round of chemotherapy approached, Ryan's blood work still showed he was neutropenic. He could not take his chemotherapy on schedule, but his numbers were getting stronger. The doctors decided to skip his chemotherapy for May and give his body another month to get stronger. As it turned out, Ryan was able to enjoy his company and his graduation without struggling with the effects of the chemotherapy.

On the morning of May 31, I got in the car and headed out on my six-plus hour trip to Chris and Andrea's home. Nonna, Poppa, and Aunt Jenti were all making the trip at the same time, all riding together. To save time, I started cutting across the back roads of southwest Missouri and northwest Arkansas hoping to catch or pass them. That was a mistake. The roads in that part of the country are extremely hilly and curvy as one is traveling in the Ozark Mountains throughout much of the region. Roller coasters were less exciting than that cross-country trip. By the time I arrived at the house, everyone else had already arrived. We had a bite to eat, and then we had the privilege of going to a Fighting Frogs T-ball game. We spent the rest of the evening playing games and enjoying one another's company. The time spent traveling caused us to desire turning in early that night. We knew the next morning was the big day and we all wanted to be well rested.

Few people knew it, but something special was planned to take place at graduation. It was something Chris had worked toward having happen, and he found out Thursday afternoon it was going to happen. We arose on Friday morning, the day of graduation and we prepared to go to the ceremony. After the ceremony, we went to a buffet for lunch and then back to Chris and Andrea's house. After we returned to their house, I wrote the following journal entry on the website in an attempt to share the emotion of what had happened during the previous twenty-four hours.

FRIDAY, JUNE 01, 2007 04:53 PM, CDT
On Thursday evening, the Fighting Frogs took the field to start the game. Before the end of the first half of the first

inning, the Frogs were down by six. Ryan led off the bottom of the first inning and his first at bat, he hit the ball down the third base line. Chris and Ryan took off down the baseline as the fielders fielded the ball. Ryan beat the ball to first and was safe at first with a clean single. The next batter up hit a shot up the middle, the second baseman fielded the ball and raced to the bag. Ryan was forced out at second. However, the Frogs were able to tie the score by the end of the first inning. Ryan was able to bat two more times and each time, he advanced the runners who were on base in front of him. He was not very happy about sacrificing, but he did what he was supposed to do. That is a tough lesson for any child to learn. The game is played as a team and sometimes we are part of a bigger game plan. We don't get all of the glory, but the team is better off. Sadly, the Frogs would end up on the short end of the score at the end of the game. They fought hard, but they suffered their first loss of the season.

Friday morning began early for us. We arrived at the high school for the ceremony. There were so many kindergarteners this year so they could not hold the graduation at their own school and accommodate all of the parents (and grandparents, aunts and uncles, etc.). The gym was all set up for the ceremony and right on schedule in the graduates marched. As Ryan's class entered, Ryan was all smiles and waved to each of us in the stands. He walked in, walked right up to the risers, and climbed to his spot on the second tier. I was moved to tears (for the first time today) when I witnessed him being able to step up the risers into his position. He did not need a hand; he did not have to stand on the floor. He stepped right into his place and stood with a smile a mile wide across his face. The first big surprise of the morning came when the principal introduced the superintendent and the superintendent introduced Arkansas State Senator, Dave Bisbee. Senator Bisbee came to present a special award. Chris had contacted the Senator's office in March and the Arkansas Senate awarded Ryan's teacher, Mrs. Vickie Kennemer, a special citation in appreciation for her outstanding dedication as a teacher. She was shocked; Chris and Andrea were called down in front of the entire gym full of people to help present the citation. I was moved to tears once again. Ryan's class was fourth on the agenda to have their diploma's awarded. Mrs. Kennemer stepped to the podium and began to call the name of each child. It became more and more apparent that she was fighting tears. When she reached Ryan's name, she choked up, but she made it through. I had tears the whole time, but then what happened next just about made me break down and weep openly. Ryan received his diploma from Mr. Martin, the principal and began his walk across the gym to his place on the other side of the gym. He walked tall and looked as proud as any graduate I have ever seen. The crowd began to clap for him and he thrust his right hand high into the air clutching his diploma. Like a conquering gladiator in Rome of old. He had fought hard and gained his victory. Diploma instead of sword, but the symbol was the same. VICTORY!!! The crowd erupted into a cheering throng. As I looked around the gym, there were tears being shed all around the room. Ryan had accomplished something that six months ago we did not know if he would ever accomplish. He had indeed won a victory.

I guess I was most touched by what happened after the graduation was over. The teachers began to clean up the decorations. There were runners across the floor and stars with each child's name on them all around the gym. As the other children were running around and playing, Ryan simply walked over to one of the runners and began to roll it up with one of the teachers. Once they got it rolled up, Ryan threw his entire body onto it to crush it down so he could carry it. After the runner was disposed of, Ryan began the tedious process of picking up the stars that were taped to the floor. Not once did he complain and to my knowledge, he was not asked to help. I think he has learned that in this life there are times you need help and times you can help. He has received his fair share of help and in this simple unspoken gesture; he did what he could do to help someone else. I think he has learned more in his young life than many adults ever learn.

We would like to thank each and every one of you who have prayed for Ryan and for our family. God has performed one miracle after another in our family. Today

was the next step forward. Please continue to remember to
pray for Ryan as he continues this journey.
    Uncle Tim

I have to admit I have never been as influenced by one person as I have been by Ryan. I never seem to stop being amazed at how mature he has been through all of the treatments and surgeries. As he strode across that gymnasium with diploma in hand, it was one of the proudest moments I have ever witnessed. I honestly don't think there was a dry eye in the entire gymnasium.

The lesson of humility that followed the triumphal reception of the diploma was incredible as well. Ryan had been through so much, yet he realized this was something he was capable of doing. Instead of sitting back and telling us he couldn't, he went out and did. The most amazing part was no one asked him to help. He saw a need and he stepped up to the task at hand. Most people are willing to help if they are asked to help, but Ryan did so without any prompting.

Senator Bisbee came toward the family, he wanted to shake hands with Chris and Andrea, and he wanted to meet Ryan personally. He had a rather incredulous look on his face when he saw Ryan was helping clean. The adults stood around talking with numbers of well-wishers. People came up and congratulated Chris and Andrea on Ryan's progress and condition and all the while, Ryan was walking around behind them picking up paper stars.

During the presentation, Senator Bisbee shared with the crowd how he and a colleague had received an e-mail from Chris describing the dedication of Mrs. Kennemer. He admitted there in the office the two Senators had both wept as they read about Ryan and about Mrs. Kennemer. They had agreed that something special should be done, so they presented it before the Senate, the commendation was approved, and the citation was issued in her honor.

It was all such an incredible event. I was overjoyed at having made the journey to Pea Ridge. I would have missed a truly blessed event if I had just heard about how it all transpired. By being there, I was able to take in the whole atmosphere. The whole time I was watching Ryan walk with his class, then stand and sing the songs with all of his heart, all I could think of was how blessed we were to be able to witness the events. A few months prior he had been so bad, but he was so much better by graduation time we knew God had performed numerous miracles. To watch Ryan triumphantly take that walk across the gym with his diploma was a Hollywood moment if there ever was one.

There had to be a pause in the calling of names because Ryan did not walk as fast as the other children did when he crossed the gym, but no one seemed to mind the extra few seconds. It also gave Mrs. Kennemer and Mr. Martin a moment to re-group their emotions and continue with the program.

Yet another life lesson was learned during the Frogs game on Thursday night. I had alluded to it in the update, but I did not go into detail on the website because it was still T-ball season and we did not want to bring about discord. In retrospect, it probably was the best decision for the team, but not for Ryan and almost not for the coach. During the course of the game, Ryan came to bat with runners on base. The Frogs were behind and had an opportunity to score a few runs. Ryan had been hitting the ball down the third base line because that placed the ball the furthest from first base. When he hit the ball down the third base line, it took a few extra seconds for the play to develop and the fielder to get the ball to first base. Those few seconds often were the cause of Ryan making it safely to first. On the play in question, the coach told Ryan to hit it at the first baseman. He wanted the play to be to first, not third, so the base runners could advance to second and third. Ryan pled his case with the coach, but the coach remained steadfast. Ryan stepped to the plate and hit the ball just as hard as he could; right down the first base line. The first baseman grabbed the ball and ran to the bag. Ryan was out. The base runners made it to second and third just as the coach had planned. The coach's plan was executed to perfection. All was right on target, until Ryan went into the dugout and began to cry.

Ryan had a tendency to want to excel at everything he attempted. In his mind, if you did not score, you hadn't achieved the goal. If you did not score a run, you weren't helping the team win. He had Nonna and Poppa, Jenti and me in the stands and he wanted to score a run to help his team. He wanted us to know he helped his team. To that point in the game, he had either gotten out, or stranded on base every time. This happened during his last at bat, in the final inning of play and he knew if he did not score a run that at bat, he wouldn't score. He had fought through the desire of his heart and he had done what the coach had told him, but it nearly broke his little heart to fail to score a run that night. When Ryan hit the dugout and began crying, Nonna nearly lost her composure. Nobody made her Ryan cry without getting an earful. Chris was very unhappy as well. I told him it was part of the game and he looked at me and said Ryan had already had to sacrifice enough. He should not have had to sacrifice his opportunity to score. Chris had played baseball for years and he knew that the coach's decision was because he was playing to win. The problem was that this was T-ball, not the World Series. Chris did not want to have Ryan sacrifice, but he did not want to undermine the coach. The family was not happy about the play, the other parents were not happy about the play, and on top of everything else, the Frogs ended up losing that night. That really made the play even more difficult to swallow.

It was a tough play and a tough decision. The coach had done what he thought best and we had to accept that fact. Ryan did what he was told, to the best of his ability, and he had been saddened by the event. His family had been very upset to see him so upset. When the game ended, we all rapidly left the park. Fortunately, there was not a big scene and by the next day, all was well once again. Ryan had not scored a run in that game, but he had won the victory. He had competed with his entire body, his entire ability and with his entire heart. Nothing more could have been asked of him.

Within that twenty-four hour period, I came to realize that victory does not always come to the one who scores the most points. Victory comes when one can give all they have to a cause they love. Ryan had done just that, both in his education and in T-ball. He had given his all, and for that reason, I believe he was the victor.

Fringe of Normalcy

Ryan had to have his blood levels checked on a weekly basis. For him to take his chemotherapy, he had to meet certain levels in several different measurements. All of the numbers were holding strong, except for the ANC. The ANC was the number that determined if he was neutropenic. He had been fighting to get his ANC number up for several weeks, and over time, the number did rebound to a level that was acceptable. Originally, the doctors had set the ANC level at 500 for continued treatment. When Ryan had trouble building up to that level, they had raised the magic number to 1000. The thinking was if his white cell count built to that level, the chemotherapy would knock it down, but not below 500. Chemotherapy had been postponed until his ANC rose.

The week following graduation, Ryan had an appointment in Little Rock. At that appointment, his ANC was 860. That reading was high enough to withstand the next round of chemotherapy, but not likely high enough to keep Ryan's ANC above 500. If it dropped below 500, the subsequent round of chemotherapy would again need to be postponed. The doctors in Little Rock made a decision they had been avoiding for a while. They did not want to decrease the dosage of the chemotherapy, but at the same time, they did not want to keep postponing chemotherapy rounds because of the low ANC. At the time of the visit, he had an acceptable ANC, so they decided to grab the opportunity and proceed with a round of chemotherapy. However, they decreased the dosage of the medicine to one-half of what he had been attempting to take. They decided it was better to decrease the dosage and treat him than to hold off treatment until his ANC climbed higher. It was a decision that would prove to be a good decision a few months later.

Andrea had some other appointments in Searcy, so she and the kids spent some time at Granny Beck's house for a few days. Andrea was able to take care of all of her extraneous appointments and they were able to visit with Carnell for a few days. Carnell had not been able to attend Ryan's graduation, but she thoroughly enjoyed getting to see Ryan and Ashtyn the following week.

After I returned home from the graduation festivities, I had to jump in with both feet to get things done. I returned home on Saturday, and my family left for Disney World the following Tuesday evening. To add to that, I conducted Sunday services before we left for Disney. That was cause enough for us being busy, but that was only the tip of the iceberg so to speak.

On Tuesday, June 5, we headed for Florida. We returned home the next week just in time for Laura and Joshua to leave again. They had to attend college orientation for Joshua. I would have gone with them, but on Friday night after we got back from Florida I had a wedding rehearsal to attend. On Saturday after we returned from Florida, I had the wedding to perform. With the rehearsal and the wedding, I couldn't go to orientation with Laura and Joshua.

All this led to a very busy schedule for us. Graduation, vacation, orientation, and a wedding all within two weeks. If these had been the only events, they would have kept us busy. However, we had even more important events happening during the month of June.

Chris and Andrea were going to be on vacation starting on June 16, and they were coming to our house on the way to Indiana. We decided to have one last open house for Ryan in Centralia. The date for the open house was set, Sunday, June 17, Father's Day. Okay, so we added guests into the mix. Still not busy enough for us I guess, because we had also scheduled Vacation Bible School (VBS) for the week following Father's Day. We were in the final stages of preparation for VBS in the times we were not tending to some of the other things happening. Now you begin to get the full picture of the month of June for me. Graduation, Sunday church services, vacation, orientation, wedding and rehearsal, visitors, and VBS. By the time everything was completed, I felt like I needed another vacation.

Surprisingly, everything went exactly as planned. I made it home from graduation, preached on Sunday and we left on vacation on schedule. We made it safely home from Florida and prepared Laura and Joshua to go to orientation. While they were gone, Jessica, Rebekah, and I worked on doing the laundry and cleaning the house in preparation for our company.

Thursday of that week, I had received word that a little girl I knew had been diagnosed with bone cancer. Her grandparents attended our church and had brought her on several occasions.

Hearing she had cancer was a shock, to say the least, but then when does one ever really expect to be diagnosed with cancer. I called her grandparents and spoke at length with them, trying to offer comfort and support. It was a topic I had become all too familiar with, while dealing with a pediatric oncology patient.

Prior to vacation, I had been preaching a series of sermons from the Biblical book of James. I had preached the series, starting at James, chapter 1, verse 1. I preached all the way up to James, chapter 5, but I did not have enough Sundays to preach that sermon before vacation. What I came to realize was God had a different timetable for the series. I was preaching that sermon on Father's Day. Ryan would be present, and he was a testimony to the prayer of faith. As I spoke with the little girl's grandparents, I encouraged them to attend the Sunday service to hear the message about praying for healing. They agreed they needed to be there to hear the message.

Friday came and with it the wedding rehearsal. Everything went smoothly and on Saturday, we had a beautiful outdoor wedding. For those of you who have never been to Illinois in the summer I can tell you that it was over 90 degrees with about 90% humidity at the start of the wedding. We had plenty of shade at the wedding site so the weather was not too much of a detriment. All in all, it was a very beautiful wedding.

Following the wedding, I went home to wait for our guests to arrive. Nonna and one of her friends, Pat, arrived and then Chris and Andrea and the kids arrived. Laura and Joshua made it safely home from orientation also, so that evening we were all together safe and sound.

We arose on Sunday morning with the knowledge that it would be another special day. It was Father's Day, which made it an extra special service. To begin the service, I asked Ryan if there was anything he wanted to say to the congregation. He walked from his seat in the congregation up onto the platform.

He took the microphone from my hand and very deliberately made eye contact with as many people as possible. "I would like to thank everyone for all of their prayers." He then handed me the microphone and walked back to his seat. There was not a dry eye in the congregation at that point.

I preached the sermon and I was very blessed to be able to use Ryan as an incredible illustration as to the healing power of God. It was undeniable, God can and does heal when there really seems to be no hope. Ryan had been to the brink of death and within just a few months, he was standing on the platform thanking a small portion of the people who had been praying for his healing for those months.

We concluded the service with a time of prayer around the altar. Anyone who wanted to come forward, be anointed, and prayed for was encouraged to do so. We did our best to follow the words of God in James 5. I have no idea how many people I anointed and prayed for that day. I was very touched by the grandparents of the newly diagnosed little girl coming to be anointed on her behalf. We prayed for her and her family that day, with the same conviction and belief with which we had been praying for Ryan.

The service was especially inspiring and people could sense God had been moving in our midst. Following the service, Chris spoke with the little girl's grandparents at length. He told them if he could ever be of service, or if they needed someone to talk to about the situation, they should call him. At the time, they were completely overwhelmed by the diagnosis, but the talk with Chris was very comforting to them. To see Ryan walk up onto that platform and offer his thanks was very beneficial to them. They had witnessed just how powerful God is that morning. The girl's cancer was not a brain tumor, but the treatment would be similar to Ryan's: radiation, chemotherapy, and surgery. It was comforting to them to see how well Ryan was doing after he had been through all of these things.

Our family ate a nice lunch together and then we gathered for the open house. Many people showed up at the open house, but there was one very special guest that came to visit Ryan. Jaylyn, the young lady who had been in the car accident the previous year, was able to meet Ryan. Her family and ours had encouraged one another through the months by posting entries on the CaringBridge guestbook pages. Chris had made it a point to leave Jaylyn and her family a personal invitation to attend the open house. She brought Ryan a stuffed orangutan that he promptly named George. We spent the afternoon visiting with all of the guests, especially Jaylyn and her mother. It was such a blessing to see Jaylyn and Ryan, who had suffered so much, sitting and laughing together.

Chris and Andrea got up the next morning and went on their way to Indiana to visit with friends. They spent the first part of the week going to visit their friends and then they came back to our house later in the week. Ashtyn and Ryan were able to attend our VBS the evening they returned to Centralia. The next morning, they got up and headed about halfway home. They spent the night in Missouri so Ryan could have a break from being in the car. He was getting tired of the traveling. They arrived back at their home safe and sound on Saturday.

It was the first week of July before Chris and family made it back to their home and updated the journal again. They had traveled in Missouri, Illinois, and Indiana before they returned to Arkansas. Ryan's ANC was a little low when he returned home, so the doctors postponed his chemotherapy for one week. By that time, he was able to take the treatment without incident.

T-ball season had concluded while the family was on vacation. By the time they returned home, it was time for them to enjoy their own VBS program. The summer was just as busy for Ryan and his family as it was for our family.

It was after they had returned home from vacation that Chris and Andrea began to notice something strange about Ryan's head. He came through the house one evening and there was a spot that had sunken inward. Chris said it looked like an overripe melon with a thumbprint. He had posted this information on the website, I did not quite understand what he was trying to explain, so I called him.

Chris told me, "The side of Ryan's head has a sunken in portion to it. Think of his head like an overripe cantaloupe. If you pushed your thumb into that overripe melon, it would leave a dimple in it. That dimple is what is showing up on the side of Ryan's head."

I thought it was a bit graphic for an illustration, but it was how he described what they were seeing.

The different MRIs that were done had shown the void created by the tumor removal had filled in with the brain as the brain had returned to its normal shape. The first MRI Ryan in November showed the hemisphere line, the line down the center of the brain, had been curved into a horseshoe shape. After the tumor was gone, the brain re-oriented itself to its correct position and the hemisphere line had straightened itself out.

In the most recent MRI, there was no indication there was a void present any longer. The lack of a void was what caused the confusion when Ryan started to have an indentation on the side of his head. The only real possibility the doctors in Pea Ridge could postulate was that perhaps the shunt in Ryan's head was drawing too much fluid out and causing a void. The doctors were concerned, but when they called Little Rock to discuss the case, there was not a sense of urgency that called for a quick trip to ACH. The course of action was to monitor Ryan very carefully and if anything further developed, it was to be addressed immediately.

Other than the indentation on the side of Ryan's head, all was going well. As the days passed, there continued to be occasions when there would be a noticeable indentation on the side of Ryan's head. It never seemed to get worse than the original indentation, but it did go away after he rested.

During the latter part of July, Chris found out that his friend Kevin had been diagnosed with cancer again. Nonna had told me about Kevin several days before Chris shared the news. It was something very difficult for Chris to accept. Kevin had been such an inspiration for us as he had undergone everything Ryan had undergone and he had been cancer free for five years. He had undergone an MRI just prior to the surgery Ryan had in February 2007. I remember him sitting with us that day and telling us he was officially five years cancer free. He had recently had an MRI, which showed no signs of cancer. Six months later, he had gone for his next MRI and it showed the cancer had returned. It was a very discouraging event because as much as Ryan had undergone we were hopeful it was all over at this point. When the cancer showed back up in Kevin, it made us all face the reality that Ryan would never be completely free of this dreaded disease. They would continue to monitor him for years to come and it could come back at any moment without any warning signs. The only way it could be determined to be present was to show up in an MRI.

Kevin began a course of treatment very quickly after they determined the cancer had returned. They did not know what the prognosis was, but Chris was calling on everyone who was praying for Ryan also to pray for Kevin.

Though Chris and Andrea had just been on vacation in June, they had a second week of vacation scheduled for the first part of August. Ryan's birthday was on August 6, and the trip was going to allow him to be at Nonna and Poppa's house on his birthday. Laura, our daughters, and I decided to make the trip to Nonna and Poppa's so we could be present for the birthday party.

Fried chicken and french fries once again abounded. One of the ironic things that happened was that Chris broke the french fry cutter we used at Nonna's house so he and I spent hours washing and cutting up potatoes while we were there. Chris was very particular about how the fries had to be cut because if they weren't cut with a certain consistency some would burn and some would be undercooked. I cut up my portion and he cut up his portion and between the two of us, we cut up and cooked about 30 pounds of potatoes over a three-day span. Nonna was not feeling well during this time and so we did most of the cooking. When it came to frying the chicken, we cooked nearly 40 pounds of chicken to go with our potatoes. Fresh tomatoes and corn on the cob rounded out the menu. Occasionally a beef roast and mashed potatoes supplemented the fried chicken and french fries. Many people ask us how we can eat fried chicken and french fries every day when we are at Nonna's house. The answer is simple. We cannot get that food any other time so we, much like camels at an oasis, stock up when we have the chance.

We had a most enjoyable day with Ryan on his birthday. Nonna, Andrea, Aunt Laura, and Ryan all went to Poplar Bluff shopping. While they were in Poplar Bluff, they met Aunt Jenti and they all went to lunch. Jenti had to work that day so she enjoyed meeting them for lunch so she could spend a little time with the birthday boy.

A whole array of family members came to Nonna's to visit and to eat. We celebrated Ryan's birthday with his cake and presents. Ryan was able to play with his cousins and he had a big day of it. By the end of the day, Ryan was tired and the indentation on the side of his head became apparent. For those of us who had not witnessed it before, we were taken aback a little bit. One time Ryan came into the room, his head looked fine. The next time he came into the room there was a sizable indentation. Chris explained this was what he had tried to describe to everyone. It did not really carry as much significance when someone tried to explain it to me as it did when I saw it with my own eyes.

Chris and Andrea stayed at Nonna's for a couple of days, and Laura, our girls, and I headed home after a couple of days as well. It was not a long visit, but it was most enjoyable. Chris and family headed from Nonna's to Carnell's house on Wednesday of that week. They spent several days there, and then Ryan had a doctor's visit in Little Rock on August 13.

During the doctor's visit on August 13, the doctor told Chris and Andrea the indentation was caused by the muscles in Ryan's head having been weakened by the radiation. When he grew tired, the muscles were not strong enough to hold their proper shape. This was not a situation that needed any further treatment; it would just happen when he was tired. During the visit, the doctor also gave Ryan the clearance to attend school. He could return to the classroom as a first grader when school began.

Ryan was very excited about getting the doctor's approval to go to school. He had finished the previous year as a homebound student and he wanted to get back into an actual classroom. The doctor warned them that when cold and flu season was in full swing, Ryan would probably need to become a homebound student again. However, for the start of the school year he could go to class with the rest of his friends.

School began on August 20, 2007, with much excitement as it does each year. Throughout the previous year there had been so many crisis moments that one year later there was even more excitement about Ryan getting to start first grade than there had been when he began kindergarten. It was nothing short of a miracle that he would begin first grade with the rest of his class.

Ryan's comprehension of his overall health was staggering. He never questioned his treatments or tried to get them stopped in any way. He wanted to get better and he knew if he did what he was told he needed to do it would help him get better. He has a medical knowledge that would put many adults to shame. He realized the importance of good hygiene and he knew all about germs.

Ryan came home from school following his first day in first grade and when his mother asked him how his day had been, he told her it had been a good day. He then went on to tell her he had gone to the nurses' office. Andrea was alarmed about the fact Ryan had to go to the nurses' office and she began to question him about what had happened.

"Ryan, why did you need to go to the nurses' office today? Were you not feeling well?" Andrea quizzed him.

"No, I felt fine. I was just thirsty," he responded.

More perplexed than ever, Andrea clarified what he had said. "You were thirsty, so you went to the nurse? Ryan, why would you go to the nurse when you were thirsty?"

"Mom, you know that little kids put their mouths on the water fountain when they get a drink. I didn't think I needed to take a chance on getting those germs when I got a drink. So, I went to the nurse and told her I was thirsty and I asked her for a water bottle," he patiently explained.

The nurse had given him a water bottle and all was well. Chris and Andrea did feel a little sheepish about the fact Ryan had caught the problem with germs in a water fountain and they had not. However, it also assured them he was aware enough of what was happening so he could protect himself in situations like that one.

With school back in session, all was going along well. Routine once more began to set into the Mondy household. However, one more special event was yet to come to pass.

Chris had been contacted about speaking at a Children's Miracle Network fundraiser that is held in August of each year. At least one professional athlete, either active or retired, attends the event to help raise funds. The organizers wanted to share Ryan's story with the people attending the event, as it was a fundraiser for all of northwest Arkansas. Since Ryan was from the area, his story hit very close to home for several people. Chris agreed to attend and speak on Ryan's behalf.

The athlete that helped in 2007 was Mr. Joe Theisman, former NFL quarterback for the Washington Redskins. Mr. Theisman had a very successful career in the NFL, playing in two Super Bowls and winning the league MVP award. As the celebrity representative for the event, Mr. Theisman had a very touching story about his own daughter being assisted by the Children's Miracle Network when she was only two years old.

When I called Chris to find out how the event had gone, he laughed about how Ryan met Joe Theisman. "Ryan was helping set candy on the tables and when he got to one of the tables, a man was sitting in his way. It turned out to be Joe Theisman. Ryan asked Mr. Theisman to excuse him as he was reaching across to put candy on the table. Ryan had not been born when Joe was playing football, but it did not take long for them to become quickly acquainted. Joe picked Ryan up and sat him on his lap. They sat and talked for a long time. At one point, Joe took off his Super Bowl ring and let Ryan hold it and try it on for size. During the course of the evening, Joe took the stage to share the story about his daughter. He shared how the Children's Miracle Network had assisted them. While Joe was on stage, he called Ryan up on stage with him. He presented Ryan with an official NFL throwback jersey from his Redskins playing days. Joe autographed the jersey for Ryan and he put the jersey over Ryan's head telling the audience what a hero he thought Ryan was."

I was impressed at the generosity of Mr. Theisman, and I told Chris so. I asked how much money the event had raised. Chris told me they had raised over $600,000 for the Children's Miracle Network that day. It had been an incredible evening and it had really touched Chris to be able to help them raise so much money. Ryan's story was indeed an inspiring story and as such, it had a way of touching people and letting them know when they donated money it was making a lasting impact on the lives of children.

A week or so passed and the local newspaper had a story about the event. It was only after the paper published the article that Chris found out Mr. Theisman had paid $1000, out of his own pocket, for the jersey he had autographed and given to Ryan. Two other jerseys had been auctioned on the night of the fundraiser. One of the other jerseys that was purchased that evening was to have been framed under glass and donated to ACH to put on display.

All in all everything was going along exceptionally well. Ryan was doing very well in school and he had not shown any signs of school being too much for him physically. He was able to go each day and stay all day long. His strength and stamina were continuing to grow. One concern started to surface was that he was getting thinner. Chris and Andrea assumed he was just growing and getting taller. They did not stop to consider he might actually be losing weight.

Ryan had another trip to ACH the second week of September and they anticipated he would go in and have his blood work and an MRI and all would be fine. Ryan had been doing so well there was no need to assume anything was amiss. The results of the tests changed all of that in very short order. Once again, we would be cast headlong into a pool of insecurity about Ryan's future.

I tried my best to keep up with the dates of Ryan's trips to Little Rock and I would call Chris on those afternoons as he was driving home so I could find out what the doctors had said at the appointments. For the past few months all had been very good information when we spoke, so when I talked on the phone with Chris after this round of appointments I was taken aback.

Ryan had an MRI performed on September 10, and when the doctor read the results, he found a bright spot that concerned him. Bright spots were indicators of abnormal tissue. The doctor told Chris he could not tell what the bright spot was with certainty. It could be a condition called radiation necrosis, which was a result of the radiation therapy. If it was the necrosis, it was not a point of concern. Another option was it could be a pooling of blood, which should heal itself and soak back into Ryan's body. The last option was the cancer had returned.

Chris left the doctor's office with a complete uncertainty about what the future held. Andrea had not made the trip to Little Rock with Chris and Ryan, so on the way home Chris called Andrea and told her the results. I spoke with him on the phone and so did Nonna while he made the journey. He was very discouraged by the time he reached Pea Ridge. He had to tell everyone he spoke with Ryan might have another tumor forming.

The doctor told Chris he wanted to schedule a more detailed MRI for the month of October. He wanted an MRI, which used a different contrast than what the hospital has, and it had to be ordered. The MRI was scheduled for October 8.

The issue of Ryan getting thinner came up at the doctor's visit also. The doctor began to wonder if Ryan was losing weight because of his body fighting another tumor. The one good report Chris did receive was Ryan's ANC count was almost 2400. A very strong number, which indicated he had a stronger resistance to colds and flu than most people had.

The possibility of a recurrence of cancer was always on the table. When Kevin was found to have a recurrence after being cancer free for five years it had been a blow to our family. It seemed as if Ryan and Kevin were connected in a way that could not be explained. When Kevin's cancer returned, it brought about a very harsh reality that it could happen to Ryan as well. With this MRI, it appeared it was more than just a possibility. The doctor would not go so far as to say it was a tumor. He said they could not tell from the MRI what was causing the bright spot they saw. He would not speculate what the spot was and he assured Chris there was equal probability for the different possibilities. All this did was to add frustration to our situation. If he had diagnosed it as a tumor, we would have moved forward. If he could have ruled out a tumor, we would have been very glad. Instead, we had a few possibilities placed before us and we had nothing we could do except wait to find out what was causing the spot.

With the spot being absent in Ryan's previous MRI, it was obvious whatever was causing the spot was moving rapidly. Not knowing what was causing the spot was bad enough, but add to that the realization Ryan had gone from cancer free to having a very noticeable spot on the MRI in a very short time span. Our concern was if it was a tumor, how much it could possibly grow before the next month passed and the next MRI was performed.

Following the MRI and discovery of the spot, Chris and Andrea began to monitor Ryan very closely for signs of a possible tumor. Before the initial cancer diagnosis, every time Ryan had a headache they attributed it to his sinuses. Following the diagnosis, they watched him very closely for any signs they had previously overlooked or attributed to sinuses. He was not having any headaches, which was a very good sign.

Ryan continued to be strong and to feel good. His numbers all looked good and that helped to pass the time with a little more ease. Had there been a major fluctuation in any of his vital signs the level of concern would have been greater. If he became sick or had headaches, it could have turned into a crisis episode. As it was, we were all concerned and praying for Ryan, but not overly distressed about his upcoming MRI. All we could do in the interim was to pray for Ryan and ask others to pray for him as well.

I toyed with the idea I would really like to be in Little Rock when Ryan went for his next MRI. Andrea could not make the trip with Chris and I just really had a burden about Chris getting the test results and not having anyone with him for support. I talked it over with Nonna and she had felt the same way. We decided I would drive to her house and pick her up on my way to Little Rock and we would go together. Then within a few hours, Nonna called me back and told me Jenti and a friend were going to go as well. Jenti did not have to work on October 8, and she wanted to be at the hospital when we got the results. I had a lot of things going on at home and so I told Nonna that if it was okay with her, I would let Jenti take her to Little Rock and I would bypass the trip altogether. I explained I just did not want Chris getting the results without having some support. She said she felt the same way and that was why she was going. I told her I would pass on the trip.

I struggled with the decision to skip the trip to Little Rock for a few more days. I just kept coming back to the point that I felt I needed to be in Little Rock when the results of the MRI were given. I also felt I needed to take my anointing oil with me, anoint Ryan, and pray for him before he went in for the MRI. I talked it over with Laura and she told me if I felt like I should go, then I should go.

I talked it over with Chris and with Nonna and decided I would make the trip. Chris started laughing when he found out I was going to make the trip. He asked if I realized it was time for the all you can eat shrimp fest at Red Lobster. It had been nearly a year since we had gone to the Red Lobster in Little Rock and stuffed ourselves with shrimp scampi. I told him that yes, I was aware of that and we made plans to go to Red Lobster on Sunday evening when we all got to Little Rock.

In October 2005, Chris and I had eaten at the shrimp fest while moving him back from Utah. In November 2006, we had eaten at the Red Lobster in Little Rock while Ryan was still in his chemical coma. Now came October 2007, and we were once again sitting at Red Lobster eating all of the shrimp scampi we could eat. On our previous trips, it had just been Chris and me, no witnesses. This year we had Nonna, Ryan, Jenti, and Jenti's friend, Bridget. When the waitress took our order, we told her we were going to eat many shrimp and every time she delivered a refill to order another refill. She did a magnificent job of keeping scampi on the table for over an hour. When it was all finished, I had eaten 190 shrimp and Chris had eaten a mere 140. He just did not have it in him to keep up with me.

Very full and very tired, we all went back to the motel. We had adjoining rooms in the motel, Chris and I in one room and Nonna and the girls in the other room. Ryan was staying in the room with Nonna and so I took my anointing oil and went to talk with Ryan. I explained what the Bible said about anointing sick people and I asked him if it would be okay for me to do that. He said he did not fully understand about it, but he said it would be fine for me to anoint him. It was just Ryan and me in the room, so I poured some oil out and anointed his head and prayed for him. I do not believe it was anything magical, but I do believe wholeheartedly that turning the matter over to God was the only real solution we had. I prayed for Ryan and then he got into bed and went sound asleep.

The next morning began a very long day. Ryan was NPO and he made it plainly clear that if he was NPO, we were all NPO with him. So, while he was in the van headed to the hospital with Chris, Nonna and I headed to the coffee shop near the motel. She was going to honor the NPO order but I did not see that my caffeine headache would accomplish anything for Ryan. I got a cup of coffee. I am not sure if it was because of the type of coffee it was or because I was supposed to be NPO with Ryan, whatever the reason I did not finish that cup of coffee, because it just didn't taste right.

We got to the hospital and waited. They took Ryan for his blood work and we waited. While Chris discussed the blood work results, we waited. Ryan had to wait to get his MRI and we waited with him. While Ryan was having his MRI, we waited some more. Finally, after six hours at the hospital we got to the point in the day for which we had waited. We got to speak with the doctor about the results of the MRI.

The MRI done that day showed that the spot, about which the doctor was concerned, had gotten smaller during the month. It had also gotten a large dark center in it, which indicated whatever was causing the bright spot was dying. The doctor told us he still could not say with certainty whether it was a tumor or radiation necrosis. At that time he told us he had "been nervous the entire month," wondering along with us what the results of the MRI would be. He told us whether it was a tumor or necrosis, it was going away. We were told if it had been a tumor trying to form, the continued chemotherapy had stopped its growth and was actually killing it. If it were necrosis, it would dissipate and go away on its own. Either way, the cause for alarm was lessening.

We walked out of the doctor's office with a spring in our step once again. There was still a cause for concern, but the doctor told us there was no need to have Ryan get another MRI the following month; he decided to wait two months to schedule the next MRI. That meant we would get to celebrate Thanksgiving Day together before we possibly had a chance to receive any type of negative results. We would celebrate the day oblivious to any future problems and we could enjoy the day together. For that, we were grateful.

Following the doctor's visit, we all went our separate ways once again. I took Nonna home, spent the night at her house, and then headed back to my home in Illinois. Chris headed straight home with Ryan. Jenti and Bridget made it home safely that night as well. We had experienced yet another moment of grace, as God had given us a favorable doctor's report and safe passage home for each one of us.

Chris had made it home late on that night after the doctor's appointment. October 9, was Chris and Andrea's wedding anniversary, so Chris had decided to take that day off from work. He was very pleasantly surprised when the doorbell rang that afternoon and UPS had a package for them. Chris had heard of a place called Worksman Cycles, which specialized in making custom-built bicycles and tricycles. Chris and Andrea had ordered a tricycle with twenty-inch wheels for Ryan and on October 9, it arrived. Ryan had loved riding his bicycle before the cancer was found. He spent a lot of time riding with his best friend, but the surgery had left him too unstable to balance on a bicycle. The tricycle gave him the ability once again to ride like the wind with his neighbor and best friend. When Ryan came home from school that afternoon, he strapped on his helmet and away the family went for a bicycle ride.

Most little boys enjoy riding their bicycles. This was just one more step in bringing normalcy to Ryan's life. The bike was not something purchased on a whim. It was very deliberate and it was expensive. It was done because it was something he needed to have to be able to enjoy riding with a cycle. We often take many things in life for granted. One such thing is the ability of little boys to ride bicycles. It is not until something like this happens that you begin to realize just how much in life we do take for granted.

Imagine for just a moment looking down at a hospital bed at a child not knowing if that child would ever awaken from a chemically induced coma the doctor had to order. If the doctor had not ordered the chemical coma, the child would have been shivering uncontrollably because of the icy blanket on which he or she was laying. Now imagine less than one year later stepping out the front door and calling that same child to come in for dinner. The child is out on the sidewalk with his or her little friends riding a brand new adult sized tricycle. Imagine the lump that would pop up in the throat as flashbacks to that picture of the child laying in that chemical coma appear in your mind. Imagine the overwhelming sense of gratitude to God for Him allowing the child to be back out riding that new tricycle. Hold on to that lump for a few seconds and imagine how incredible of an experience it was for Chris and Andrea when Ryan received that tricycle.

With the positive report from the doctor, Ryan breezed through the month of October. He had his tricycle and loved going outside to ride it every opportunity he could.

As the month of October 2007, came to a close, the anniversary of Ryan's diagnosis and surgery loomed on the horizon. It was not an anniversary we really wanted to celebrate, but at the same time, it was something we could not avoid. It turned out to be a very emotional week.

Halloween brought the anniversary of Ryan dressing up and going trick or treating at his dad's office, just before he became critical. In 2006, he had collected candy from his dad's co-workers; however, he did not get a chance to eat it before he was rushed in for surgery. By Halloween 2007, Ryan was once again able to collect candy from his dad's co-workers. This time he got to eat it. Ryan's costume for Halloween 2007, was none other than a very fitting Superman costume.

Since the calendar shifts every year it is not possible to have an anniversary of an event on the same day of the week as it was the previous year. Ryan had been diagnosed on Friday, November 3, 2006, and had been airlifted to Little Rock that same evening. Some of the events we began recollecting were based on the day it happened and some were on the date the events occurred. On November 2, 2006, Ryan had a headache and Chris had forgotten to stop and get a refill on an antibiotic. If he had remembered the antibiotic there is no telling what would have happened.

I called Chris on Saturday morning, November 3, 2007, and talked with him for a while about how Ryan was doing and we talked about what had happened during the previous year. I asked if he cared if I wrote another journal update from my perspective. He welcomed the opportunity. I wrote an update on Saturday morning and hit the button to update the website and it had wiped out my entry. I had spent a long time writing that update and it was gone. I decided I would not update that day. My daughters had a piano recital, in which they were both to perform. I had missed that same recital the year before, because I was in Little Rock waiting on the surgery to be completed. I decided I did not have time to re-write an update because it was too close to the time we had to leave.

We went to the recital and it happened to be at the local Hallmark store. While we waited for the girls' turns to play, we wandered around the store. I had decided to skip the journal re-write until I ran across a

Christmas tree ornament from *Bee Movie*. I stood there in Hallmark with tears in my eyes as everything that had happened the previous year on this day came flooding back.

One day several months prior to Ryan's diagnosis, Ryan had gone to work with his dad on a Saturday. That Saturday, Mr. Jeffrey Katzenberg, CEO for DreamWorks Animation, had been at the office as well. Mr. Katzenberg had spent a considerable amount of time that day talking with Ryan about the movies Ryan liked and disliked. Mr. Katzenberg had asked Ryan about some particular DreamWorks pictures and Ryan had given him input from a child's perspective. Ryan went on to tell Mr. Katzenberg about why he liked some movies that competitors of DreamWorks were making. Mr. Katzenberg had been very taken with Ryan and his maturity.

A few days after Ryan had been diagnosed and had been through his surgery. Mr. Katzenberg had heard about his little friend and had sent him a care package. In the care package, there were numerous items related to DreamWorks pictures. One of the items in the package was a promotional item from *Bee Movie*. None of us had ever heard of *Bee Movie*. The reason I was so touched when I saw the ornament in the Hallmark store was the movie had just opened in theaters. It opened on the weekend of the one-year anniversary of Ryan's diagnosis and surgery. That ornament brought flashbacks of Ryan laying there in that bed and how we wondered about all of the items included in the care package and also wondered if Ryan would ever be able to see those movies when they were released to the public. He had survived those days and he was indeed able to watch the movies Mr. Katzenberg had wanted him to know were being released in the future.

Ryan had a doctor's appointment on Monday, November 5, 2007. It was the one-year follow-up to Ryan's original diagnosis and surgery. I decided the doctor's report would be a fitting conclusion to this book. I waited through the rest of the weekend and on Monday afternoon I called Chris as he was headed home.

On November 5, 2007, Ryan had blood work done. His ANC count was over 3100. He weighed in at fifty-two pounds and was just over forty-eight inches tall. He was strong and healthy.

God had given us Ryan for at least one more year. We had no idea how long his journey on this earth would last, but then again we did not have any assurance of how long each of us would live either. We had spent the past year drawing strength from one another and from the people who had been praying for Ryan and for the rest of our family. God had been merciful and He had been gracious. We had been granted strength and we had been given an opportunity to try to encourage others who were undergoing difficult times. I believe that is why I felt so compelled to share Ryan's story with the world. His is a story of triumph over tragedy and hopefully, it is a story that will lift the spirits of everyone who hears about him.

I had originally planned, as I said previously, to conclude the book with the one-year anniversary doctor's visit. I wanted to conclude the book, get it published, and then encourage everyone to keep up to date via the website. Well, I found out that publishing is a very slow process and it does not happen quickly enough to accomplish what I intended.

As the months continued to pass following that doctor's appointment, more events continued to happen. I chose to continue writing as long as I could to give the very latest information in the closing pages of these memoirs.

On November 14, 2007, Ryan celebrated his one-year anniversary of being removed from the ventilator. Chris had wanted to re-watch the movie *Cars* with Ryan to commemorate the anniversary of their watching it in the PICU. However, they were not able to watch the movie that night. Ryan had joined the Cub Scouts and on that night, Ryan was receiving his first Tiger Beads as a Tiger Cub.

A few days after getting the Tiger Beads, Ryan went to the brand new McDonald's restaurant grand opening in Pea Ridge. Ronald McDonald was present at the opening. It was an incredible scene from what Chris said. Ryan had met Ronald at the RMH in Little Rock the previous December. When they entered into the new restaurant, it was the same Ronald and he actually remembered meeting Ryan in Little Rock. When Ryan had met Ronald the first time, it had been at ACH. Ryan had already relocated to the Ronald McDonald House. When he saw Ronald at the hospital, they had engaged in a conversation.

Ryan told Ronald, "You know what, Ronald, I am staying at your house."

"Well that's great," Ronald responded.

"So will you be home for dinner tonight?" Ryan had asked Ronald.

At that point, Ronald couldn't stop himself from laughing. When Ryan and Ronald met in Pea Ridge, Ronald remembered that exchange and still thought it was quite funny.

Ashtyn's birthday fell on Thanksgiving Day in 2007. We had all gathered at Nonna and Poppa's house for the holiday, so the kids were all present to help Ashtyn celebrate her birthday. Throughout the day, we reminisced about how we had spent Thanksgiving Day in the hospital cafeteria the previous year. It was so much better being at

Nonna's house for the big Thanksgiving meal. We tried to keep count throughout the day and the best we could tell, somewhere around thirty people ate at her house sometime during the day. During the afternoon, several of the kids decided to hold a dance contest. Ryan jumped right in the middle of the contest, until his dad got onto him for getting too rowdy without his brace on his leg. There was no lack of desire in the boy, just a little loss of mobility still.

It was incredible how much better Ryan's mobility had become since I had seen him playing with his cousins in August. I had seen Ryan at the hospital in Little Rock in October, but there were no other kids around for him to play with on that trip. When he got together with other kids, one would never have suspected all he had undergone.

The day after Thanksgiving, Nonna, Andrea, Chris, and I all went shopping for bargains. We were in Wal-Mart before 5:00 a.m., and we didn't have to worry about getting back to the hospital this time. The kids were all safely tucked into bed at Nonna and Poppa's house and Poppa was there to care for them while we shopped.

Chris shared the information with us that Ryan's picture had made it onto the rear cover of the Children's Hospital ACHiever magazine. It is a magazine that gives information about the hospital and includes several inspirational stories. The magazine is published quarterly and for the Fall 2007 edition, Ryan and Joe Theisman are on the back cover. I checked the hospital website and they have a digital archive of all of the past ACHiever magazines, from Winter 2003 until Summer 2007. The edition with Ryan had not been posted at the time of this book being written. If anyone is interested in seeing the magazine, check the ACH website and search for the ACHiever link. Hopefully in the future, the issue will be archived and one will able to see the picture of Ryan and Joe Theisman.

Ryan had an MRI between his Thanksgiving and Christmas visits to Nonna's house. The MRI was done on December 3, almost exactly one year from the day he began his radiation and chemotherapy treatments. The results of the December MRI were identical to the results of the October MRI. When the doctor reviewed the results of the two MRIs side by side, there was no change. He indicated to Chris that the spot was most likely due to radiation necrosis. His reasoning was if it were a tumor, it would have either grown or shrunk. By the spot staying exactly the same size, it was most likely not cancer. That gave us all an emotional boost when we heard.

While Ryan and Chris were at the hospital for his December MRI, they cut through the play area on the third floor. Chris said when they neared the area, someone he knew asked if they were going to stay for story time. Chris had not planned on it, but as he looked around, he realized something exciting was happening. He was given a release form that he had to sign to stay in the area. As they waited, Chris looked around and saw some of the upper executives from the company he worked for standing around also. After a short wait, they found out what was happening. The First Lady of Arkansas, Governor Beebe's wife, had come to the hospital to read a story to the children. Her reading was carried on the closed circuit television channel of the hospital so any child who could not get to the play area could still hear the story. Once the story was completed, toys were passed out to all of the children in the hospital. That was why the executives were present. That company had donated all of the toys to be distributed.

We all returned to Nonna and Poppa's house for the Christmas holiday season. Chris and family arrived a few days before I was able to get there. Our menu once again centered around fried chicken and french fries. One night before we got there, Nonna had made meat loaf. Ryan was very upset because he understood he had been promised Nonna's fried chicken would be available every night. He was very disappointed and apparently threw a fit. We were not there, as I said, but that did not happen again the entire time we were there. After that night, there was fried chicken and fench fries at every evening meal, regardless of what else was being fixed.

Typically, we open gifts at Nonna's house on Christmas Eve. As soon as we had eaten our holiday meal, the gift opening started in earnest. The kids opened gifts for close to an hour, and they loved every gift. Ryan was near me while he was opening his gifts and I asked him what he liked best about Christmas. He looked to me and said very childlike, "I like that we get to celebrate Jesus' birthday." I had not expected that, but I guess I should have expected the unexpected out of Ryan.

One of the most moving events of our holiday stay of course involved Ryan. Jenti's friend Bridget, who had gone to Little Rock with Jenti in October, brought her fiancée, Buddy, to the house. Buddy is a soldier and had recently been deployed in Iraqi. Buddy had undergone some scary encounters in Iraqi and Ryan had become a pen pal to Buddy. Ryan drew pictures to send Buddy and in one particular picture, Ryan had drawn a winged creature in the background. When Chris asked Ryan about it, he said it was Buddy's guardian angel. Ryan and Buddy had never met face to face, until the day after Christmas. Buddy came in and Ryan had his back to Buddy.

Buddy walked up to Ryan and introduced himself. "You must be Ryan. I am Buddy, the one you have been writing to the past several months."

Ryan laid his toys down, held out his hand, and shook Buddy's hand, "Well Buddy, it is a pleasure to finally meet you."

The two of them sat down and talked for a bit, and they had a great time doing so.

The next morning Chris, Andrea, and the kids headed south to Granny Beck's house for a few days and then they returned to Little Rock for a New Year's Eve check-up. When Ryan went to the clinic on December 31, he was forty-nine inches tall and weighed fifty-four pounds. The doctor started increasing his chemotherapy amount when he began taking the round for January. He moved from a 100 mg dose to a 140 mg dose. He took the complete round of chemotherapy, without any negative side effects. The week following the completion of that round saw his ANC over 2300, so he was apparently able to tolerate the higher level of chemotherapy.

Over the Christmas holidays, I had heard the latest update on Kevin. The doctors had tried a variety of methods to treat his cancer, but nothing seemed to be working. Then after the first of the year, I found out his medications were switched and he had started getting better. It would appear God was not finished with Kevin yet. Our prayers continue to be that God would be there every step of the way to help Kevin through the "valley of the shadow of death." Little did we know how much Kevin's treatment and Ryan's would once again be linked together.

The Greatest Miracle

With the passing of the holiday season, school began back in earnest. During the month of January 2008, Ryan began to show increasing signs of having difficulties with his schoolwork. When he practiced his material at home, he would do well. When he would take tests at school, he would not do as well. Or, perhaps, the situation would reverse itself. Ryan might begin very strongly in his mathematics and poorly in spelling or reading and when the time for his tests arrived, he would do well in spelling or reading, but poorly in math. Ryan had a check-up scheduled toward the end of January, so Chris decided to wait until that visit to talk about Ryan's problem rather than make a special trip to Little Rock to discuss the matter.

After Ryan struggled for a little over a week, it was time for the trip to ACH. During the check-up, Ryan had an MRI and his normal round of blood work. The blood work all appeared normal, with an ANC of 3600, and the MRI did not show any further irregularities. No mention was made of the spot that had been present since the September 2007 MRI. Chris assumed that the spot had not changed because the doctor did not mention it. While at the hospital, Chris spoke at length with the medical staff about Ryan's trouble in school.

The response to the situation was to schedule Ryan for a visit to a neuropsychologist, who would determine what course of action was to be taken. Chris learned that radiation therapy commonly causes this type of memory loss in a cancer patient. The ideal outcome would be to have the testing performed and determine if the problem was a result of radiation, typical seven-year-old forgetfulness, or some other reason. Once the testing had been performed, a therapy course would be determined to decide how to re-train Ryan how to learn.

Chris returned that evening to Pea Ridge with an explanation as to why Ryan had been having troubles learning. The answer was rather simplistic in nature, Ryan's body was continuing to show the effects of the radiation. Following the testing, he would have a new learning plan and life would return to the previous state.

Ryan returned to school the next day and life continued as they awaited the neuropsychologist appointment. As the week continued to unfold, Ryan began to have more trouble walking. He became more prone to falling. The following week began to show other signs that something more serious was wrong.

Speech became slurred and Ryan began to forget more things. He used his left hand less and less. When he used the left hand, it had virtually no strength. On Friday of that week, Ryan fell down at school and bumped his head. By the following Monday, he had begun to drool and the left side of his face began to sag a bit.

Chris and Andrea talked with the doctors at the local hospital and they advised them to contact ACH immediately for advice. When they contacted the doctors at ACH, the advice was to take Ryan to Little Rock immediately so he could be checked.

On February 11, Chris and Ryan returned to ACH and Ryan was admitted to the hospital. A few tests were done that day, but they were inconclusive. More tests were scheduled for the next day, including another MRI.

Prior to an MRI, Ryan always had to be NPO, without food OR drink, at least eight hours before the test. For some reason the nurse delivering his morning medications did not realize he was NPO. She gave Ryan a glass of orange juice to take his medicine. Once he finished off the glass of juice, his clock was reset and the MRI had to be rescheduled for late that afternoon. Finally, around 4:00 p.m. Ryan was taken to have his MRI performed.

Following the MRI, Ryan was given his evening meal tray. On the tray was a snack cake. Ryan picked the cake up and looked at his dad, "This has caramel in it doesn't it, Dad?"

"Yes, Buddy, it has caramel," Chris responded.

Slightly forlorn, Ryan looked to Chris and said, "I can't eat it then."

"Why not?" Chris wondered aloud.

"I gave up caramel for Lent," Ryan simply explained.

When I heard the story, my heart broke for the poor little guy. With all of the struggles he had battled through, he still had the fortitude to keep his promise to abstain from caramel for the Lenten season. He had not had any food in almost twenty-four hours, and only one glass of orange juice during that time. In addition to the restriction on food, Ryan had been awakened every two hours through the night to check his vital signs. Thus, he was very tired. He ate the other food on his tray, but left the caramel filled cake lying uneaten.

The next day, Jenti called the hospital gift shop and had a goody basket sent to Ryan's room. Ryan anxiously dug into the basket and pulled out a Snickers candy bar. Again, he looked to his dad and said, "Snickers has caramel in it doesn't it Dad?"

"Yes it does," Chris tenderly replied. It was difficult to see Ryan not getting to eat the food he knew Ryan would really enjoy. Chris refrained from making excuses though and allowing Ryan to eat caramel. Ryan had determined to give caramel up for Lent on his own and Chris respected that commitment.

Suddenly, Ryan's face brightened. "Snickers is covered in chocolate isn't it?"

"Yes it is. Why?" Chris asked.

"Because you gave up chocolate for Lent, so my candy bar will be safe until I can eat it," Ryan chirped.

Ryan's optimism had never waivered. The caramel incident fully illustrated both his determination and his optimism. He would not cave-in and eat something he had willingly decided to abstain from eating. He was not discouraged about the abstention; he was optimistic it would still be there when his commitment was completed. I was humbled by Ryan's attitude once again.

The results of the MRI done that day showed a spot near Ryan's brainstem. Chris found the doctors had noted the spot on the MRI in January, but they had not mentioned it. They were going to monitor the spot in subsequent MRI's and see if it changed. They also informed Chris that the spot of concern on the September 2007 MRI had disappeared. That spot had apparently been radiation necrosis.

A spot showing up in the January 2008 MRI had not been a major concern because the previous spot indicated radiation necrosis was a strong possibility for the new spot. The level of concern was low following the January MRI. However, with the increase of negative symptoms, the level of concern rose. The latest MRI confirmed the spot was present.

Scar tissue and swelling made it very difficult to determine if the spot had increased in size between the two latest MRIs. The doctor ordered another test, one that was a special form of MRI that caused necrosis to show up one way and cancer to show up a different way. This was very new technology and it allowed for a definitive diagnosis of the spot.

As the test was basically another MRI, Ryan was once again NPO. This time the test was performed earlier in the day. We waited throughout the day with no word about its result. Finally, on Friday, February 15, we got word from the doctor. The cancer had returned.

We had been warned for over a year this was a possibility, even a probability due to the type of cancer. It was very difficult to hear the words that the spot was a new tumor. The fight had returned. Ryan's symptoms had been developing, not because of a learning problem, but because a tumor was growing and placing pressure on his brainstem once again.

When Ryan had entered the hospital earlier in the week, the doctors had determined the best course of action would be to begin giving him steroids to reduce the swelling in the area of the spot. They assured us both necrosis and cancer were equal possibilities, and that either would cause the swelling Ryan was experiencing. They had begun the steroid regimen early in the week. Steroids would be given for either condition to minimize swelling. The diagnosis of cancer did not alter the need for steroids, but it meant steroids would not be the only medication Ryan needed.

Chris discussed the situation with the doctor. The oncologist told Chris that during the previous year progress had been made in developing new chemotherapy treatment for this type of cancer. The doctor was very optimistic the new chemotherapy would be effective for Ryan. He explained there were two medications that would be given as a "chemotherapy cocktail." It would be administered through an IV. It would take six hours to administer, and then there would not be any further treatment for two weeks. After the two weeks, another dose would be given. This cycle would repeat for eight weeks, then they would perform another MRI to see what the tumor was doing.

If the treatment worked, great. If it didn't work, they would re-address the course of treatment after the next MRI. He went on to tell Chris they had found it possible to use a variety of chemotherapy drugs to treat this type of cancer, but in some patients they had to continue altering the "cocktail" and adding or subtracting different elements to get the right combination for a given patient. The thing he wanted to make most clear to Chris was there was a good chance one combination would work to destroy the cancer again.

Not wishing to waste any time, the doctor had Ryan transferred to the oncology ward in the hospital and the chemotherapy was administered that afternoon. They wanted to keep Ryan in the hospital for a few days to make sure he did not suffer any ill effects of the new chemotherapy before they sent him home.

As it was on Friday, Andrea picked Ashtyn up from school and they made the trip to Little Rock that evening to see Ryan. Andrea had remained home to allow Ashtyn to attend school through the week. They had already planned to be in Little Rock that weekend, before Ryan started having problems.

Every year the Ronald McDonald House and ACH each have fundraisers to help provide funds for the upcoming year. Chris and

Andrea had been asked to speak at the RMH fundraiser, "The Chocolate Ball," Saturday night of that week. The staff had grown very fond of Ryan during his stay at the house the previous year and they knew his story touched the hearts of everyone who heard it.

During the week, ACH had its annual fundraising drive. One radio station broadcast the event on the air to help raise funds. The previous year, the station had dubbed Ryan's voice over a song and played it on the air. While the song was played on the air, the switchboard lit up with calls from people wanting to contribute to ACH. With Ryan in the hospital during the 2008 fundraising drive, he ended up in the lobby while they were broadcasting. The announcer was extremely touched by Ryan and the track from the previous fundraiser was re-aired. Once again, the switchboard lit up. By the time the fundraiser was completed, the hospital had raised over $300,000 in their efforts.

Chris had a goal in mind. When he had spoken at the "Will Golf for Kids" fundraiser for the Children's Miracle Network in August 2007, that event had raised over $600,000. The two fundraisers combined meant that Ryan's story had helped raise over $900,000 for the two charities. Both of the events had record levels of giving and many people associated with the events believed Chris' sharing of Ryan's story had helped. Chris determined that if they could help the McDonald House raise $100,000, again a record amount for them, Ryan's story would have helped generate over $1,000,000 to help other children.

Saturday night rolled around and Chris spoke to the crowd gathered for the ball. As was generally the case, there was not a dry eye in the auditorium. Before the evening was completed, generous contributors had given enough to reach the overall $1,000,000 goal Chris had set for them. One man asked Chris how he could possibly stand in front of all of those people and share such painful memories with them. Chris simply told the man it was far easier sharing the memories than it had been to live through them.

The rest of the weekend passed with the family in Little Rock. Ashtyn was out of school the following Monday, so they didn't have to rush back to Pea Ridge on Sunday. However, on Monday, Chris decided it was time for him to return to work. He took Ashtyn back to Pea Ridge. She returned to school on Tuesday and Chris returned to work.

On Tuesday, I called Andrea to see how Ryan was. We talked for a long while. I asked her several questions about Ryan's upcoming weeks and she said she had talked to the doctor about most of those that morning. It was not their regular doctor, but an intern. She, as well as I, was surprised when he could not answer several of her questions. The reason, we found out, was that much of the treatment Ryan was undergoing was cutting edge technology. The second test that had been done to determine whether the spot was cancer or necrosis was such a new technology that the intern had only read of it recently and had never had any experience in the test being performed. The chemotherapy regimen was the same story.

After Andrea and I spoke at length, a therapist came to get Ryan for therapy. We finished our conversation so Andrea could give her attention to the therapist. I was rather surprised then a few hours later when Nonna called me and told me Ryan was going home that afternoon. The decision had been made while Ryan was gone to therapy. So, after just a little more than a week in the hospital, Ryan went home.

The expectation was Ryan would be homebound for the remainder of the school year. However, when he was released from the hospital, the doctor gave him clearance to go back to school the following day. The following day happened to be picture day at school, so Ryan was excited about going to school to be in his class picture.

Ryan made it to school the day his picture was to be taken, and was in the class picture. He also had his individual picture taken; however, by lunchtime he began to wear down physically. The nurse called Andrea to the school to take Ryan home.

On the way home with Ryan, Andrea had to pick-up Ashtyn's Girl Scout cookie order, which contained over four-hundred boxes of cookies. After getting the cookies and taking them and Ryan home, Ryan took a nap. Once he had rested, he wanted to help sort cookies. So, that evening they began an assembly line to sort and bag boxes of cookies. Ryan was responsible for four kinds of cookies and he set about unboxing the cookies and placing them in the appropriate orders. He was not able to use his left hand very much, but he did use his left arm to help hold him up while he reached across his body with his right hand to get the cookies out of the box.

The following day, Ryan was once again too tired to attend school. He stayed home with Andrea and rested. Andrea called the doctor's office in Little Rock to find out if she needed to change anything. The doctor's office recommended she increase the steroid level by fifty percent. Ryan was still not at the level they wanted him to be with his speech and mobility. Actually, Ryan's speech had slipped so low he was nearly unintelligible when he spoke. He reached a point where his communication became little more than pointing and grunting. He easily became frustrated because people could not understand what he was trying to say.

On Friday morning, Ryan began taking a third dose of steroids each day. It had been one year to the day since Ryan had undergone the second surgery to remove the tumor. We had gone for months with Ryan being cancer free. Now we were once again in the middle of the battle for life.

As the weekend passed, Ryan continued to physically decline. On Saturday, Chris cooked fried chicken for them to eat. Ryan was excited about eating fried chicken, so when it was cooked, he began to eat. Andrea removed the chicken from the bone and broke it into bite-sized pieces. As Ryan began voraciously eating the chicken, he became choked. He began gasping for air. Apparently, he had a small channel open in the food lodged in his throat because he continued breathing in gasps until Andrea could remove the bulk of the food from his mouth and throat. While Andrea worked on removing the food, Chris called 911. The rescue team arrived at the house and checked Ryan. When they arrived, Ryan's air passageway was obstruction free; he was safe for the time being.

On Monday, February 25, Ryan still was not improving in his speech or mobility. He awoke that morning and while Andrea began dressing him, he cried and said he did not want to go to school. Andrea assured him he did not have to go to school that day. A few minutes later, as Andrea continued to help him get dressed, he began crying again. When Andrea asked why he was crying, he said he did not want to go to school that day. Andrea became alarmed, as they had just had that conversation a few minutes earlier. Ryan did not remember the conversation.

Andrea called the hospital in Little Rock to see what she should do. Ryan had become completely listless, not able to hold himself upright as she helped him put his shoes and socks on that morning. He slumped over and lay on her shoulder as she helped get his brace on his leg and then his shoes. His speech had not improved over the weekend of increased steroids. By all accounts, he was getting weaker and Chris and Andrea were very concerned. The doctor's office advised her to drive Ryan to Little Rock as quickly as possible. They packed a bag and got on the road by mid-morning. I spoke with Andrea as she traveled and I could tell she was very concerned. I began praying for Ryan and started sharing the concern with others through the CaringBridge website. We had been asking people to pray for him and I had begun a movement to ensure we still had prayer support in all fifty states. In just over a week, we had a representative from every state committing to praying for Ryan. I sent out the call for more prayer.

After Andrea and Ryan arrived in Little Rock, Ryan began undergoing several tests. One MRI was performed and a shunt function test was performed. Ryan was not sedated for the MRI, he was so listless that he lay perfectly still during the test. Then we waited for the diagnosis.

Ryan was admitted to the hospital that evening and we did not have any idea how long he would remain in the hospital. Chris had remained at Pea Ridge with Ashtyn. Andrea had packed a bag with the knowledge they could be gone for a week or more. Tuesday morning dawned and there was no improvement. Ryan was continuing to get physically weaker. His right side started getting weaker as well as his left. His left was virtually non-functioning and his right was very weak when he tried to move around at all. The doctors decided that until they had the test results, they would put Ryan on a full liquid diet to keep him from choking again. We did not get any results from the tests that were performed when Ryan had arrived at the hospital. All we could do was wait and pray.

Tension was nearly palpable when we spoke on the phone to one another. Wednesday afternoon, I called Andrea to see if she had gotten any test results. The only test result Andrea received was the shunt test result. Based on the test done on Monday, the shunt was functioning perfectly. There was no kink or crimp. Fluid from the brain was draining just as it should. No report on the MRI though. And so, we waited.

I was torn as I tried to write website updates each day. I knew there were many people faithfully reading the website. I started tracking the numbers and it seemed every time I wrote an update between four and five hundred hits were recorded. I wanted to let people really know how serious Ryan's condition had become, but I did not want to alarm them. I struggled because it was very difficult to remain positive about the news I was getting from the hospital. We were not getting the test results very quickly. In addition to the lack of information, it appeared Ryan was getting worse.

One comment Andrea made greatly concerned me. During one conversation with her, she said something about an increase in the size of the tumor could be the cause of the problems. The doctor did not say the tumor had increased, but speculated an increase in size could account for everything.

Then something strange happened. The doctors did not give Andrea any MRI results, but they told her they were going to increase Ryan's therapy regimen to two times a day. They also planned to do a "swallowing test" on Thursday. They wanted to see if they could determine why Ryan was choking on his food.

Jenti called me on Thursday morning. She was nearly in a panic about why we had not heard the results of the MRI. As I talked with her, I felt God was giving me some insight. The doctors had not told us the MRI results, but they had suddenly become more aggressive in their approach to therapy. I speculated an increase in therapy meant the doctors were more concerned about Ryan's physical ability and strength than the MRI results. I told her I assumed the MRI had not shown any significant results and so they had not spoken about the test. Little did I know how wrong I was.

Thursday of that week, Ryan underwent the "swallowing test." They gave him food, which had barium in it. When he swallowed the food, they could monitor the food's path down Ryan's throat. What they determined was his throat muscles were not strong enough to transfer food from his mouth to his stomach in one swallow. Food traveled part way down his esophagus and then would stop. The next bite of food would stack on top of the previous bite. Eventually, the food was pushing itself down into his stomach, but it caused him to choke in the process. He was also experiencing a lack of feeling in his throat and so he could not tell when the food stopped partway down. As they monitored him, they would tell him to "dry swallow" which meant he was supposed to swallow without anything in his mouth so the muscle contractions would transfer the food in his esophagus to his stomach. Then he could take the next bite and continue eating.

The test helped them to realize that one of the worst things for Ryan was liquid. Liquids passed too quickly through his windpipe and as such, they could aspirate and get into his lungs. It he got liquid in his lungs, it could cause pneumonia. A thickening agent was the solution. Before Ryan drank any liquid, the thickener was added to it. The thickener would slow the liquid down so Ryan wouldn't get it into his lungs.

Friday happened to be a unique day. It was February 29, Leap Day. Ryan had been in the hospital all week long again and his symptoms appeared to be about the same, or maybe a little worse than when he entered the hospital.

For some reason, Rebekah, my youngest daughter, got out of school early on that day. I headed across town to get her after school. As I drove across town, I had to stop at an intersection. As I sat at the intersection, I heard, "Things are going to change." I looked beside me to make sure I was alone in the van. I did not hesitate to believe God was speaking to me, but I didn't really know about what He was speaking. It wouldn't take long for me to find out what was going to change.

I retrieved Rebekah and we went home. I heated something for my lunch and I had just sat down to eat. I had not eaten more than a few bites when my phone rang. It was Laura, I talked with her for a minute or so, and I pushed my food around my plate with my fork while we talked. As we talked, call waiting beeped and indicated I had another call. I looked at the caller ID and it was Chris. I told Laura I needed to go so I could find out what Chris wanted. He should have been at work in the middle of the day and I was concerned about why he was calling.

"Well, we finally got the results of the MRI," he started.

"OK, what did the test show?" I continued pushing my food around my plate.

"The tumor is gone!" Chris beamed.

I dropped my fork and asked him to repeat what he had said.

"The tumor is gone," he continued. "There is a necrosis spot on the brainstem. The necrosis is what is causing all of the problems with Ryan's speech and loss of mobility."

"That's amazing," I interjected.

"Some might call it a miracle," Chris quipped.

"I guess so," I concurred. "By the way, I got my manuscript back from proofing today. I guess I have to rewrite the end now."

"Is that a problem?" Chris questioned.

I assured him it would most definitely not be a problem to re-write the conclusion.

I set about writing the new ending to this book. My heart soared as I penned the words that Ryan's cancer was gone once again. I rushed to get the newly finished ending to my proofreader and she made corrections. I hurriedly compiled the sections of the book and promptly sent it to the printer. I ordered two proof copies, one for me and one for Chris. Then we waited for the proof copies to arrive.

During the second week of March, the proof copies of the book arrived, both at my house and at Chris' house. We eagerly began to read through the work looking for any further corrections or changes that needed to be made. Chris read the entire book in less than two days. He made a few comments about things which needed to be corrected and my wife Laura read our copy of the book and made corrections to ours as well.

As self-publishing a book is a multi-step process, I continued with the aspects which needed addressed while others were doing the final readings. Once I had my part done, I sat about making the final round of edits to the manuscript. I spent numerous hours editing and correcting the work. By mid-March, I had received my ISBN, the barcode that is assigned to all books sold in any commercial marketplace. I needed to add the barcode to the title page of the book and insert the barcode on the cover image. On March 18, I was running my spell-check program one last time to make sure I had not created an error in the editing process. Since I was rushing to finish that day, I had taken my computer to the dentist's office to edit while I waited on my children to see the dentist.

While I was at the dentist's office, my phone rang. Caller ID said it was Chris calling. I thought it was odd for him to be calling; it was the middle of the afternoon. I stepped into the foyer so I could hear him clearly.

"What's up?" I asked as I answered.

"Andrea just called me from Little Rock," he began very slowly.

The tone of his voice was all wrong. There was a pronounced hitch in his voice. Immediately my mind flashed back to that November 3, 2006, phone call that had rocked my world. "Surely not," my mind screamed.

He proceeded very slowly, "The oncologist just spoke with her. He was concerned about Ryan's lack of progress in therapy. The doctor had a CT scan done today to see how the necrosis was looking."

"And what did it show?" I interrupted.

From the sound of his voice I could tell that there had to be tears falling as he slowly continued, "Another tumor has been found. It must have been under the necrosis layer when they told us the last tumor was gone. This tumor has spread beyond the necrosis area and is growing rapidly. The doctor said that since the cancer was growing and Ryan has been taking the chemotherapy, the therapy will not work. There is nothing they can do for Ryan now."

I stood in the foyer, stunned beyond words. My mind reeled, what was I supposed to say? "Chris, I am so sorry," finally flowed from my lips. "What are you going to do?" I gently asked.

"I am almost home now. I have to pick up some bills and our suits then I am headed to Little Rock," he quietly spoke.

I nearly lost my composure when I heard him say he was picking up their suits. In that instant, I knew that he did not anticipate Ryan returning home with them. He was getting their suits for Ryan's funeral.

"Does Mom know yet?" I gingerly asked.

"No, I called you first," he responded.

"Would you like for me to call her for you?" I offered.

"If you wouldn't mind, I would appreciate it. I don't think I can talk to her right now," Chris sounded a bit relieved.

"Okay, I will let you go so you can get your stuff together, I continued, "I will call Mom for you. Is there anything else I can do for you? Do you want me to put this information on the website?" I queried.

"I can't think of anything else right now," he slowly responded. "Don't put this on the website yet. I want to get to Little Rock and spend some time with Andrea before we make the news public. I don't want people reading the website and calling her while she is there by herself."

"Just tell me when you want the information put up and I will take care of that for you also," I assured him. "Call me back if you want to talk some more."

"I will," he managed. "Thanks for all your help. I will talk with you later," and he hung up the phone.

I stood in the foyer for a few seconds. Rebekah stuck her head out the office door and told me the dentist wanted to speak with me. I went to confer with the dentist about Joshua's teeth. Jessica still was in the chair in the other room, so I still had some time before we could leave the office. I took Joshua back to the waiting room and asked him to pack my computer in my bag and to keep an eye on Rebekah. "I have to go to the van so I can make a phone call," I told him. I didn't want to break the news about Ryan to the kids until we had gotten home. I knew firsthand that getting that news in the dentist's office was not preferable.

I walked out to my van so I could have a quiet, private place to break the news to my mother. I prayed that God would give me the words to say when Mom answered the phone. I was not sure how I was going to break the news to her, but I knew I had to tell her, not ask for Dad. Chris had done that with the initial phone call in '06 and it didn't seem to help soften the blow. I made up my mind that I would just be straightforward with her and break the news as gently as possible.

I called her cell phone. Four rings and then to voice mail. I couldn't leave a voice mail. I decided to call their house phone. Much to my relief, Poppa answered the phone.

"Hello," he answered.

"Dad, I have something I have to tell you and it is not good," I began.

"What's up?" he hesitantly asked. I could tell that this was all eerily familiar to him.

"I just talked to Chris. Ryan's cancer is back. The doctor said there is nothing more they can do," I spewed.

Pausing for a second, all Poppa could say was, "Oh, no."

I continued, more deliberately this time, "Chris didn't think he could handle calling you and Mom, so I offered to make the call for him. He is on the way home to get his stuff and then he is going straight to Little Rock."

Poppa and I talked for a few minutes, but I didn't have much more information to share at the time, so he agreed it would be best if he broke the news to Nonna rather than me trying to call her cell phone again. As soon as we finished our conversation, I called Laura and broke the news to her. I was rapidly beginning to lose the sense of reality. I began to grow numb all over as I talked. The more times I recounted the news, the more it seemed to be impossible. I could hear the words coming out of my mouth as I broke the news to people, but it was almost as if I didn't believe the words that I was speaking.

I went back into the reception area to wait for Jessica. As I sat and waited, Nonna called me. I stepped back into the foyer and we talked for a while. She had called Jenti and told her. I asked Mom if she had called Chris. She said that she had not. She wanted to give him some time before talking to him. I agreed that was probably best. She had called me because she wanted to know what my plans were going to be for the coming days.

Our kids were on spring break during that week. That was why they all had dentist appointments that day. They were all out of school so we were trying to get medical and dental appointments all scheduled for that week. Our intent had been to travel to Nonna and Poppa's house on Wednesday night and then Nonna and I were originally scheduled to go to Little Rock to spend some time with Ryan and Andrea at the hospital. Nonna was calling to see if I was going to alter my schedule. As we talked, I told her I had to wait until Laura arrived home from work so we could make plans. I told Nonna that I would call her back once I knew more details. Our conversation ended with both Nonna and me in tears. I composed myself and went back into the dentist's waiting room once more. I was getting some odd looks as I had been in and out of the waiting room several times by this point. Rebekah told me that the dentist wanted to confer with me about Jessica's teeth.

I spoke with the dentist once more and finally, after a little more than two hours, we were mercifully finished at the dentist and we headed home. Laura called me to let me know she was on her way home from work and told me that she would like to be present when I broke the news about Ryan to the kids. I agreed to wait, and so I waited.

After Laura arrived home, we talked for several minutes about how to break the news to the kids and we talked about what we would do in the coming days. Finally, we called the kids together and broke the news to them. They had been curious about why I had spent so much time out of the waiting room, but they had not felt they needed to press for details. When we explained the situation to them, they all shed some tears. As we discussed the situation, we began to hammer out the plan for the coming days. We decided that we would leave the next morning and drive to Little Rock to spend some time with Ryan while there was still time. I called Nonna and Jenti to tell them of our plans and they arranged to go at the same time. I called Chris and told him of our plans and during that conversation he told me to update the website. He had arrived in Little Rock and he was at Andrea's side. It was time to let readers of the website know what had been discovered.

On the morning of March 19, we drove to Jenti's house, where we gathered with Poppa, Nonna, and Jenti to go to Little Rock. We drove through rain the entire day it seemed. The weather report was for rain and more rain. As it turned out, several sections of the highway we traveled to Little Rock were closed, due to flooding, the day after we arrived at the hospital.

When we arrived, we were able to go directly to Ryan's room. Chris and Andrea had spoken with the doctor again and they were out of the room when we arrived, speaking with the childcare specialist. They were in the process of sharing the news with Ashtyn.

The staff at the hospital was well aware of Ryan's prognosis by the time we arrived. The doctor had told them that anything Ryan wanted, he was to have. They never said a word about how many visitors Ryan had at any one time. They had placed him in one of the largest rooms on the ward, to help accommodate his many guests. As I walked into Ryan's room that day, I saw a tired, weak little boy in the bed.

As we all walked into the room, his eyes followed the entrance of each person. He looked around at Nonna, Poppa, Jenti, Laura, Joshua, Jessica, Rebekah, and me. It was as if suddenly something was confirmed in his little mind. Chris and Andrea had decided not to tell Ryan that he was dying, they didn't want him to be afraid or anxious. They wanted him to enjoy his last days and hours. When we all walked into the room, I believe Ryan had a confirmation that he was not going to survive this round of the fight. He didn't seem scared; he seemed peaceful. He enjoyed the hugs and kisses from everyone that came into the room. I looked around at the visitors that were already present when we arrived. There was Granny Beck (Carnell), Uncle Steve with glasses, Aunt Iris, and Ryan's cousin Katherine. The room was rather full, as one might imagine.

I had not seen Ryan since Christmas at Nonna's house. When I had last seen him, he was jumping and playing with the other children. That was not the Ryan I saw when I entered the hospital room. Ryan was virtually paralyzed on his left side. He had lost the ability to smile, because he had lost control of the muscles on the left side of his face. He could not speak as he had lost the use of his vocal cords. He had numerous IV lines running to his portacath port. They had removed the tube from his nose and his food supply was administered through his port. He seemed very tired, and when he responded, it was slightly delayed. He could nod or shake his head and he could point with his right hand. Though his communication was limited, he let us know what he wanted.

He had two cards with pictures on them. They were his "wants" and "needs" cards. He would hold his hand up to get our attention. Someone would ask him if he had a want. If the answer was yes, they showed him that card and he would point to what he wanted. If the answer was no, they would show him the needs card and he would point to what he needed. If he wanted something that was not on either card, communication became a series of questions that he would either nod his head yes or shake his head no. It was sometimes difficult to figure out what he wanted, but eventually, we would understand what he desired.

As we sat and talked, Ryan watched TV much of the time. He had the speaker beside his ear, so he could watch the TV and hear what was being said. We talked to him and he would respond, but if anyone stepped between him and the TV, he would point his finger at them and then point for them to step to the side so he could see his program. He made it very clear that he did not want his TV viewing interrupted.

Though he was limited in his physical movements, he was still completely aware of what was happening all around him. He had not lost his sense of humor in the least. He could not laugh aloud; however, his whole body would shake when he began to laugh. The harder he laughed, the more his body shook.

Ryan had several plush *Cars* characters, and some of them spoke when they were shaken or pushed. Ryan loved to have the one that shouted "Ouch" thrown at people. He would point to the car and then his target, usually someone who was not paying attention to him. It was quite startling to be hit with a flying car that suddenly shouted "Ouch." The target would typically jump from being startled and Ryan's little body would shake as he laughed at the response.

After we arrived at the hospital on that Wednesday, we spent the remainder of visiting hours at the hospital. There was a steady stream of visitors who came to Ryan's room that evening. Off-duty staff members, Ronald McDonald House personnel, family, friends, and the list continued. As news of Ryan's condition spread, so did the list of people who came to visit. As visiting hours ended, we left Chris and Andrea with Ryan and the rest of us went to our respective motels. Ashtyn came with Laura and me so she could stay with Rebekah.

Big plans were in the works for Thursday. Ryan's portacath had to be de-accessed after seven days. It would then be re-accessed for the next seven days. Thursday was the day that the switch was scheduled to take place. The doctor wrote a pass for Ryan to leave the hospital while he was de-accessed. Chris had recently bought a new truck, a big Toyota Tundra, painted bright red. Ryan had not gotten to ride in the truck because he had been in the hospital since his daddy had gotten the truck. He had heard about it, but he had not even seen it. That day, Ryan was dressed in his Ryan Newman shirt and Ryan Newman autographed cap, and he went for a ride in Daddy's big red truck.

The trip was a short trip, around the block to the Ronald McDonald House, but to Ryan it was a taste of freedom. The weather was beautiful, hovering around 75°F and sunny. Flowers were beginning to bloom and the sweet smell of spring was in the air. Ryan had a mission he needed to complete and they took the opportunity to complete it on the outing.

The Ronald McDonald House had adopted Ryan as their symbol of hope. They had actually created a wall of hope which featured Ryan's picture. When we arrived at the RMH, we all entered to see the wall. It had the word HOPE in big, gold letters at the top of the wall. Beneath the letters were two large pictures of Ryan from January 2007, when

Ryan had been living at the house, taking his chemotherapy and radiation treatments. The third picture on the wall was a large picture that had been taken in January 2008. We all stood in tears as we saw the tribute to Ryan on the wall, and then Ryan completed his mission to the house.

While Ryan had the tube down his nose, liquid nourishment was pumped through the tube to feed him. He realized that the tabs on the containers were the same type of tabs that he had been collecting from soda cans to donate to the RMH. The donated tabs were a fundraiser for the house. Ryan and Ashtyn had spent many hours prompting people to save their tabs for the RMH. When Ryan realized his food cans had those tabs, he insisted the tabs be saved for the RMH. On his outing that day, Ryan took that bag of tabs to the house so they could turn them in to get money to help support the house. Even in his weakened physical state, Ryan had the heart of gold that everyone had grown to love. Given the opportunity to go for a ride in Daddy's new truck, Ryan wanted to go and share with the staff at the RMH so they could gain funds to help support the house.

Leaving the RMH, Chris, Andrea, Ashtyn, and Ryan went for one final ride around the streets near the hospital. The windows were down as they cruised around the neighborhood. Ryan was so weak that Ashtyn had to sit beside him and help hold his head steady as they traveled. Ryan loved the ride though. When he returned to the room and was back in bed, he nodded as vigorously as he could when asked if he had a good time on the outing. He was exhausted, but he loved it.

Ryan took a nap and during the afternoon, the nurse re-accessed his port. Awakening from his nap, a sparkle was in his eyes again. He was so happy that afternoon. His family still surrounded him. He laughed and laughed as we told funny stories and jokes. The greatest source of enjoyment for him came that evening when he wanted to have all of his cars lined up on his tray so he could see them all.

Aunt Laura dutifully sat about lining his cars up and when she finished, she asked Ryan if they were all right. Ryan shook his head and pointed at them. She moved a car or two and then asked again. Again, he shook his head no. For thirty minutes, Laura worked to get Ryan's cars lined up exactly as he wanted them. Everyone was helping her arrange the cars, but she didn't know the names of the different characters. As they would mention a name, she would pick up different cars and ask if it was the named car. Ryan thought this was hilariously funny. His body shook repeatedly as she struggled to identify each car. When it was all to his satisfaction, it was obvious that he did indeed have a pattern. Like cars had to be beside one another. Something had to be put in the front and back of the lines of cars so they wouldn't roll off the tray. Eventually she had the cars just as he wanted them, then he wanted the tray pulled up as close to him as possible so he could look at them. He didn't have enough strength to play with them, but he very much enjoyed looking them over.

We left the hospital after a busy day. Ryan was resting comfortably and we knew that he needed his rest, so we left a couple of hours before we had to that night.

Sometime during the day on Thursday, Laura found herself at the store. She found two *Cars* posters and she bought them for Ryan. On Friday morning when we arrived at the hospital, she gave them to Ryan. He was excited about the posters, but after the first one was hung, we realized he had no more wall space. Not knowing what we would rearrange, we came up with the idea to hang the second poster on the ceiling right above Ryan. He thought that was a stellar idea. Chris climbed up on one side of his bed and Andrea climbed up on the other side. As they stretched to hang the poster, Ryan laughed and laughed the entire time. He thought it was quite funny to see his parents standing on the furniture, stretching and straining to hang the poster and at the same time keep from falling. They got the poster on the ceiling and Ryan lay in the bed looking up at the poster. Then he wanted his bed raised so he could see the other poster on the wall.

The therapists came to do therapy with Ryan, and I believe they used it as an excuse to see him. Five different therapists came in as a group to work with Ryan that day. While they worked with Ryan, I stood to one side next to Chris and we talked.

"Have you told Ryan the cancer is back?" I asked.

"No, but I think he knows. He saw an angel last night," Chris said very matter-of-factly.

"Oh, really," I speculated.

"About midnight last night," came Chris' reply.

"How do you know he saw an angel?" I wondered aloud.

"He was pointing at something and we asked him if it was an angel. He nodded his head that 'Yes' he had seen an angel standing in the room," Chris simply stated.

We had been told by the child services staff members that it was not uncommon for children to report seeing angels shortly before they passed away. As Ryan had progressively gotten weaker during the previous days, it was a logical question for Chris to ask when Ryan began communicating something different than he normally tried to tell the people around him. I stored that information away, and began to wonder how much longer Ryan would be with us.

The doctor had told us that we could take Ryan out of the hospital if we wanted to, but the effort needed to get him ready to leave made Chris and Andrea re-think that opportunity. They decided they would take him down to the lobby, to the play area that was there. As the day passed, Ryan slept more than the previous two days. By mid-afternoon when he awoke from a nap, we asked if he wanted to go for a ride in his chair. He shook his head no. I asked him if it was too much effort to get ready to go and he nodded yes. He was too tired to mess with a ride.

During the earlier conversation with Chris, I asked if he had told Ryan that it was okay to stop fighting so hard. He had told me that he indeed had told Ryan that it was not necessary to fight. Child services had warned Chris and Andrea that some children will not stop fighting until they are given the assurance of their parents and caregivers that it was okay for them to quit. Chris and Andrea had given Ryan that assurance. And so, everyone decided that it really was not worth the trouble required to go for a ride. He was tired and he wanted to rest. We let him rest.

Friday evening, Ryan got our attention and signaled that he wanted to watch the big TV. In his room there were two TVs, and he had been watching the little one. It was more comfortable for him to lie on his left side so he watched the TV on that side of the room. He had decided he wanted to lie on his other side, which turned him toward the bigger TV. Chris and I carefully positioned Ryan so he could see the TV, then he began to motion toward his cars and the TV. Chris asked if he wanted to watch *Cars* the movie on the big screen. That little head began to nod with a very definite yes. He wanted to watch his favorite movie.

The movie was available on-demand, so Chris began the movie. Everyone was out of the room except for Chris, Ryan, and me. As we watched the movie, Chris came to parts of the movie that he found funny and we watched that segment three of four times. We laughed at the segment and then we realized that Ryan was actually watching us and laughing at us instead of the movie. We continued to watch the movie and I found a scene I thought was uproariously funny. Again, we re-watched that segment a few times and Ryan laughed at us.

As evening approached, Mames came back to the hospital. She brought Granny Beck with her. With a room full of visitors, Mames asked Ryan if he wanted her to sing *Little Bunny Foo Foo* for him. He again vigorously nodded affirmative. Mames sang the song, performing all of the motions and appropriate facial manipulations. Ryan did not stop laughing through the entire song.

More off-duty staff came by Ryan's room to visit. Some were on-call, some were leaving for the weekend, and some were just coming to work for the weekend shift. The parade of visitors did not slow down and by Friday night, Ryan was completely exhausted. We left a bit early again that night so he could rest.

On Saturday morning, we arrived back at the hospital. When I arrived, Chris told me that they had given Ryan some morphine that morning. He had started having a headache. This was the first pain medication he had needed. He began to move a bit more, not always an expected or intended movement it seemed. The doctors and nurses came through frequently to check on him. Many of Chris' co-workers, as well as more family members, were scheduled to visit as it was the weekend.

A little after 10:00 a.m., Ryan received a very special phone call. His NASCAR hero, Ryan Newman, had been contacted and asked to call Ryan. Actually, plans had been made for Ryan Newman to visit Ryan on the next Thursday, but as Ryan seemed to be getting weaker, the plans were altered and a phone call was made sooner than Mr. Newman could get to Little Rock. When Mr. Newman called, I had stepped out of the room. I tried to let everyone else know that Ryan was going to receive the call so that we could stay out of the room and make it a little quieter for the call. Mr. Newman called and they put him on speakerphone for Ryan. As Mr. Newman talked, Ryan would nod or shake his head in response to Mr. Newman's questions. The call was short, as it is difficult to carry on a one-sided phone call, but it meant a great deal to Ryan. As the many guests arrived throughout the day, Ryan beamed as his dad told everyone that Ryan had gotten a call from Ryan Newman.

By mid-morning, the room was once again of visitors. One friend of Chris' brought Ryan a stuffed alligator that had a music box in it. If the button in the alligator's leg was pushed, the alligator began to swing its tail and open its mouth. It sang *See You Later Alligator* while thrashing about. Any time Ryan saw this woman, she would say to him "See you later alligator," and Ryan would respond "After while crocodile," as they parted ways. Ryan absolutely loved the alligator, and he motioned for them to put it under his blanket beside him. Then we realized what he wanted. He had the alligator placed so when people leaned over the edge of the bed to give him a hug or a kiss, they would inevitably hit the button on the alligator and it would begin thrashing around under the covers and start singing. Ashtyn came into the room and leaned in to give her brother a kiss and sure enough, she hit the button. As the alligator began to move and sing, Ashtyn jumped a foot or so off the ground in astonishment. Ryan laughed harder than I had seen him laugh in the previous days. He thought that was an absolutely wonderful practical joke, and I had to agree. It was extremely funny.

Shortly after noon, I called Chris and Andrea out into the hall. I discussed my need to leave with them. Sunday was Easter and I really felt that I needed to return home as I had an Easter message that I felt God wanted me to share with the congregation. They both assured me that they agreed I needed to be back in my pulpit for Easter Sunday service. About 1:00 p.m., we said our goodbyes and gathered around Ryan's bed for a parting word of prayer. The room was packed with visitors and as we gathered there, I sensed that Ryan was not long for this world. I hated to leave, but I felt that as much as I wanted to stay, I needed to go.

Jenti and Poppa were planning on leaving also, but the flooding that had occurred during the days we were in Little Rock prohibited them from traveling the roads they needed to use to get home. Jenti leaned in and asked Ryan if that was God's way of telling them they needed to stay in Little Rock. Very eerily Ryan looked up at Jenti and nodded his little head yes. She nervously laughed it off and leaned back. We hugged, kissed, and then left the hospital.

We drove for about three hours and Jenti called my cell phone. She was very upset. They had re-positioned Ryan in bed and he immediately began to have respiratory distress. He began choking and couldn't breathe. I told her where we were and asked if we needed to return. She said she didn't know and hung up the phone.

We pulled over on the side of the road and I called Chris.

"What is going on?" I began the conversation.

"We re-positioned Ryan and he began choking. We used the suction and cleared a bunch of stuff out of his throat. He is breathing much better right now," Chris assured me.

"Do I need to come back?" I poised the question so that he could not generically tell me to use my own judgment.

"I think he is alright for now. I don't think it's time yet," he slowly responded. "There isn't anything you can do here anyhow. You go on home and share the message that God gave you for tomorrow morning."

"Okay, if you are sure you don't need me to come back now. I will be back as quickly as I can get here after the morning message," I concluded and hung up.

It took about four more hours for us to get home, but just as we were pulling into the driveway, Jenti called again. She was hysterically weeping and trying to talk at the same time. I couldn't understand much of what had been said. I got out of the car, went into our house, and immediately called Nonna.

"He is gasping for air every breath," Nonna wept. "Chris and Andrea are talking with the doctor now. I will call you back when we know more."

I sat in my chair and began searching for flight options back to Little Rock. I could not make the drive in less than seven hours, but I was finding it took longer than that to fly because of the schedules and layover times. I felt trapped.

A little later, Chris called me, "The doctor said Ryan is gasping for air because his primal brainstem has taken over. He is posturing now. The doctor said that Ryan's body has involuntarily taken over his breathing and heartbeat. His conscious brain is no longer in charge; it is the body's survival instinct that has taken control. One of his pupils is fixed and dilated and the other is very slow to respond. The swelling has shut the conscious brain out."

"Is there anything they can do?" I asked, knowing the response.

"The doctor said they can give him some anti-anxiety medicine to help him relax. The medicine will help him return brain function to the conscious brain instead of being a reflex. He warned us that if we don't give him the anti-anxiety medication, he could continue for several days in this condition. If they help him relax, he may go much quicker, but he will not be struggling the entire time." Chris brokenly explained.

Though I knew what his response would be, I went ahead and asked, "So which option are you going to chose?"

"I told the doctor not to let him suffer," Chris choked out the words.

"He's gone isn't he?" I suddenly wondered aloud.

"No, he is receiving the medicine and he is breathing easier for now," came Chris' reply.

"If he makes it through the night, I will be there as fast as I can get there after I preach in the morning," I assured Chris.

"I don't think he will be here that long," Chris simply stated. "You are the only one who can do any good right now, and that is to present the message God gave you. All we can do is sit and wait."

After hanging up from that call, I spoke with Nonna once again. I was ready to get back in the car and rush back to Little Rock that night, but she assured me that they had discussed the situation and Chris was adamant that I not be called back. It seemed that they had known several hours earlier that Ryan wasn't likely to survive the night, but Chris did not want me to be there and miss the opportunity to share the message God had given me for Easter.

Before we ended the conversation, Nonna gently asked me, "Do you want me to call you when he is gone?"

"Yes, I will keep my phone by me all night," I told her.

It was after 11:00 p.m. by the time I got off of the phone with Nonna. I decided that if I was going to be able to preach the next morning, I needed to get some rest, so I went to bed.

A few minutes before 2:00 a.m. on March 23, 2008, I received the call from Nonna. Ryan had passed away at 1:49 a.m.

I spoke with Nonna just a few minutes before she said they were going to their motel to try and get some rest. I told her I would talk with them later in the day. I went back to sleep and slept until about 6:00 a.m. when Chris called me. He said they had cleared all of Ryan's belongings from the hospital room and they had waited for the funeral home to take his body. He wanted just wanted to talk for a few minutes, so we talked. He told me a bit about the final few hours, and then he told me to get some more rest and he would talk with me later.

Easter morning was perhaps the most difficult sermon I ever presented. These people were an extension of my family and they had been praying for Ryan for months. Many of them had met Ryan during the open house at the church the previous June. I had felt that I needed to be at church that morning to share the Easter message with them. Now the time had come to share, and I didn't know how I would manage as tears continued to flow from my eyes as I thought about Ryan.

Our congregation typically averaged in the mid-60's, but on Easter morning, there were over one hundred people present. I began the service with the announcement that Ryan was gone. I told them that my family was in Little Rock and they were hurting. I explained that I would like to have been with my family, but I felt that God had a special message for them that morning, and I was going to be faithful to present that which He gave me to share. I encouraged the congregation to approach praise and worship time with the knowledge that God had brought me back to preach the message and had brought each of them into the service to hear the message. I wanted everyone to be aware that if God had brought us together that morning, He indeed had something for them to hear.

We had a very inspirational song service and the congregation truly seemed moved as they sang songs about our Risen Savior. Then it was time for the message. When I stood to speak, God removed the anguish that I had been experiencing and He gave me the ability to share from the bottom of my heart. When the message was finished, I gave an altar call for people to ask Christ into their lives. We had two altars in our sanctuary and both of the altars lined with people. We prayed with everyone at the altars, but I still didn't feel as if we were finished. I gave a second opportunity to come to the altar and more people came to pray. It was a glorious morning; people who seldom hear the Word were there and heard that God loved them enough to send His Son on their behalf. I preached about the stone in front of the tomb being rolled away and how there was no stone that God could not remove, no stone that could separate us from Christ. I truly believe every word I preached that morning, and people's lives were changed because I was faithful to preach, even when my family was hurting.

I spoke with Chris later in the day and he shared some of the arrangements for the funeral. As it was Easter Sunday, they did not have all of the details worked out, but they did know the funeral would be on Wednesday of that week. I told him that since it would not be until Wednesday, we would wait to travel on Tuesday, as there were some loose ends we needed to tie up at home.

We spent Monday in a bit of a haze as we rushed to tie up all of the loose ends. Joshua had to return to college. His spring break was over and he needed to go back to class. I shared that information with Nonna and Chris and they both assured me that they understood. They were glad Joshua had gotten to see and say goodbye to Ryan the previous week.

Tuesday morning, we got on the road and drove to Searcy, Arkansas, where the funeral was to be held. I had not been to Searcy since Christmas 2006, when we shared the day with Granny Beck. That had been a joyous gathering; this time it was not so joyous. We arrived that evening in time to gather with the family for a meal at Carnell's house. While we waited for the meal, the pastor who was to preach the funeral came and sat with the family for a while. He wanted to gain more insight into the family's state of being, and see if there was anything he could do to assist us. During his visit, I learned a lot about what had transpired during those final hours after I had left Little Rock.

Shortly after we left that day, one of the staff had gone to a local mall and gotten the Easter Bunny. They had gotten in the staff member's car and gone to the hospital. The bunny changed into the costume in the room adjacent to Ryan's so that a mob didn't form as a huge Easter Bunny walked through the main entrance of the hospital.

Andrea took bunches of pictures of Ryan as the Easter Bunny entered his room. In the pictures, it is obvious that Ryan was quite surprised by the Bunny's arrival. The Bunny stood an impressive eight feet tall and towered over Ryan's bed. Ryan was so happy that the Bunny had found him. While the Bunny stood by Ryan's bedside, Ryan began to get choked. They moved quickly to clear his airway with suction and finally got him comfortable once again. The Bunny retreated from the room and broke down in tears.

After the Bunny left, more family and friends had arrived to visit. As the hours passed, Mrs. Kennemer, Ryan's kindergarten teacher, called. She had been in Florida and she was not going to get back to Arkansas for a bit. She called Ryan and she too was put on speakerphone so Ryan could hear her. He had been very pleased to hear from her, and he understood everything she said.

Chris continued to share details of the evening with us, and he choked up a bit every once in a while. "The last person that Ryan responded to was Nurse Valerie."

The night Ryan was admitted to the hospital in 2006, Nurse Valerie had cared for him the entire night. Following surgery, Ryan was awake for a very brief time before they sedated him. During that time, Nurse Valerie had cared for him. The following Saturday when he awoke from his chemically induced coma, Nurse Valerie was once again on duty. Following his second surgery in February 2007, Nurse Valerie was once again on duty to care for him. She had been with him from the start.

Chris continued explaining to the pastor, "The ICU doctor had been called when Ryan started struggling that evening. Apparently, he let Nurse Valerie know that Ryan was in trouble. She rushed up from the PICU to see him. She gently told Ryan that he was her brave boy and that it was okay for him to stop fighting. She told him goodbye, and then she left. Shortly after she left, we re-positioned him and he began having trouble breathing again. He never responded to us again after that."

We sat and talked for better than an hour while the meal was being prepared. We shared about the laughter and about the tears. We shared our meal that evening and then we went to the funeral home for a private family visitation. As we entered the funeral home, we immediately saw bright floral bouquets that had been sent. Chris and Andrea had decided that they would recommend memorial donations to the Ronald McDonald House of Little Rock in lieu of flowers, but many people had wanted to send flowers anyway. Ryan's favorite colors had been bright, vibrant colors, much like his personality. His absolute favorites were orange and blue, and that was reflected in several of the floral arrangements. Orange was a predominate color in the flower selections as well as ribbons and other trim items.

As we approached the child-sized casket, our attention was drawn to the image of Ryan Newman's car that had been stitched into the lining of the lid. Ryan was dressed in his Easter suit and in each hand he grasped his favorite *Cars* characters. He looked very serene and he did not show the ravaging effects of the cancer. The image of him in that little casket might seem disturbing to some, but it brought peace and closure to our family. He had fought so bravely and so hard for such a long time that to see him resting like that was calming to our hearts. He had battled to the very end. He had actually done his PT/OT regimen on Saturday. He didn't back down. He did what he was asked until the very end.

It was growing late after we finished at the funeral home, so we went back to the motel. Chris had several co-workers who were driving in that night to attend the funeral, so we sat in the lobby and visited with them as they arrived. Finally, I became too tired to wait with them any longer and I went to my room to get some sleep.

Wednesday, March 26, 2008, we held Ryan's funeral. It had been one week exactly since we had made the previous trip to Little Rock to see Ryan. It seemed surreal that we had found out on Tuesday, March 18, Ryan's cancer was again growing. He passed away on March 23 in the early morning. Five days from receiving the news, Ryan was gone. As this day dawned, we would lay to rest the body of Ryan.

The day began by having another meal provided for the family. We gathered at the church for lunch. The funeral home in Searcy was not large enough to hold the number of people expected to attend the funeral, so the public visitation and the funeral had been scheduled at the church in which Andrea had been raised. As we were served lunch, the body was delivered from the funeral home along with the numerous floral arrangements. The number of floral arrangements had more than doubled since we had been to the funeral home the night before.

At 1:00 p.m., the public visitation began. During the visitation, a memorial photo slideshow played on the projection screens. As people started to arrive for the visitation, the sanctuary began to fill. I had counted the number of seats earlier in the day; we preachers like to get a good feel for how many are in any given congregation for some reason. The sanctuary seated three-hundred and fifty people. By the time the 3:00 p.m. service began, nearly three-hundred of those seats were filled.

Family, friends, co-workers, ACH employees, and McDonald House staff members, all made the journey to Searcy for the funeral. Several teachers from Ryan and Ashtyn's school, as well as the school's principal, attended the funeral. A number of Ryan's friends and classmates, along with their parents, had made the sojourn as well.

There were four preachers involved with the service at the church and a fifth preacher who helped at the graveside. I was one of the preachers to speak and I simply began with, "I am Uncle Tim." At that point, people started reaching for tissues and sobs could be heard across the congregation. I shared with them from my heart before I shared a prayer with them.

I shared about how in November 2006, I mentioned to Chris that I wondered why. Chris immediately knew I had not seen the movie *Cars*. I asked how he knew that. He had replied, "In *Cars* you find out that 'why (y) is nothing more than a crooked little letter that never did much of anything.'" I shared how that conversation had changed my outlook, and how it had made me realize it was better to move forward than to be stuck asking why.

I went on in my comments to share that I had stopped asking why and I had moved on to asking for peace in Ryan's passing. As I led the prayer, I prayed God would give peace to everyone in the congregation. I concluded my prayer, the next pastor shared Psalm 23, and the next pastor shared his sermon. It was a beautiful sermon and it brilliantly captured the spirit of who Ryan was.

The service ended and the mourners filed past the casket to say their final farewells to Ryan. As the hundreds of people left, almost every one of them stopped to give Chris and Andrea a hug. As the last of Ryan's friends left the sanctuary, the family was given a few minutes to say our final farewell to Ryan. Then they closed the casket and removed it to the awaiting hearse.

Walking out the doors of the church, I was immediately struck by how beautiful the day was. Sunny and about 75°F again. Once more we could smell the freshness of spring. We drove to the graveyard and the line of cars was so long that we could not see the last car in line from our place toward the front of the line.

The pastor that spoke at the graveside reflected on how many groups of people were present that day because they had been touched by one very special little boy. Every group that had been represented at the church had followed to the graveyard. The pastor spoke for a few moments, then we prayed together, then it was over.

We stayed around talking with the people who had attended, but with many of them traveling long distances to get to Searcy, most people did not stay around very long. It was finished and we left the graveyard, leaving behind one small coffin, containing the remains of one extraordinary boy.

The first day I arrived in Little Rock following the news that Ryan was losing the battle with cancer, I asked Chris how he was doing. His response gave me some insight to his frame of reference. He told me that on that night back in November 2006, he had prayed that God would do what He would do. He told God that night that if Ryan was to be taken, Chris' one request was that Ryan not suffer. Chris went on to share with me that he believed that God had loaned him sixteen months with his little boy and he could not be angry with God because He had been so faithful in caring for Ryan that entire time. I asked how Andrea felt. Chris assured me that she completely agreed with him; God had been good, and they were not going to turn their backs on Him when things got painful.

After that conversation, I knew that Chris and Andrea would be greatly sorrowed at the loss of Ryan, but they also possessed the hope of spending eternity with him. In retrospect, I believe God honored Chris' request to the very end. Ryan did not have any pain medication until the Saturday morning before he passed away. He began to develop a headache as the swelling continued to increase, so they continued to monitor his pain and if he was hurting, they gave him medicine to help with that pain. Chris and Andrea had five last days with Ryan and in those days they laughed, shared, and loved the entire time. Ryan did not lose his mental capabilities until the very end. He knew everyone until after Nurse Valerie said goodbye. He laughed all afternoon that last Saturday and he was surrounded by those that loved him.

Ryan may have only lived for a little over seven years, but in those seven years, he accomplished more than most people do in ten times that many years. He taught people about courage. He shared his wit and his laughter. He loved those around him and he was loved in return. His story has inspired people to do the right thing. He became an advocate for the hurting and the sick, though he himself was very ill most of that time. He was the face of hope, courage, and inspiration for hundreds, nay, thousands of people who knew him. He fought the battle until the very end, and then he peacefully went to sleep and didn't awaken again in this world. Even his passing was extraordinary. He fought to remain in this world until Easter morning. When he went to sleep in this life, he was a tired, sick little boy. When he awoke in eternity, it was on Easter morning. Imagine, spending your first day in Heaven at the feet of Jesus on Easter Sunday.

Just to illustrate how special this event was, here is a tidbit of information I found out a couple of days before Ryan passed. Easter can never occur earlier than March 22. The last time that date was Easter was 1818. Moving to March 23, that last time Easter occurred on that date was 1913. It will not occur as early as March 23 again until 2160. Ryan fought the battle to reach Easter morning; I believe he wanted to spend it with Jesus.

And so, one may wonder about the title of this last chapter, *The Greatest Miracle*. I believe that of all the miracles God performed in our family during Ryan's life, the greatest one was giving us the strength, grace, and peace to let go of Ryan. I was blessed to be part of this amazing little boy's life, and as I have done my best to share his story with each person who reads this book I hope his story inspires them. I hope people are inspired to love their children more. I hope they do more with their lives than let them pass by without merit. I pray that nothing like this ever afflicts any reader of this book, but if you know someone who is battling, don't let him or her give up hope. When hope fails, despair reigns.

I shared with Chris the desire different people expressed in wanting us to continue maintaining the CaringBridge site. They told me they wanted to see how the family continued to adjust to life after Ryan. I told Chris that I believe people see something in our family they desperately want in their own lives: HOPE. Most people who have heard Ryan's story have been inspired by him. They have seen that our hope was not placed in whether or not Ryan was healed. People have realized that our hope was something greater. Our hope lies in the promises of the Bible, one of which is that we will be re-united with Ryan, along with a host of other family and friends, because we have trusted Jesus Christ as our Lord and Savior. In this troubled day and time, people need a source of hope. Our hope is in Jesus Christ. We miss Ryan very much, but we do not despair. We believe God is still in control and we believe that we will one day get to be with Ryan, except it won't be the little boy who is battling cancer. It will be the glorified little boy who was able to spend a special Easter at the feet of Jesus.

As I type these final thoughts, my heart aches because I miss Ryan. Tears often fill my eyes, making it difficult to see the screen. I look forward to seeing Jesus and Ryan in Heaven one day, but until that day, I will continue to reflect on these *Memoirs of Miracles*, which God has granted us.

www.ingramcontent.com/pod-product-compliance
Lightning Source LLC
Chambersburg PA
CBHW020609270326
41927CB00005B/243